Losing Our Way
in Healthcare
The Impact of Reform

Losing Our Way in Healthcare

The Impact of Reform

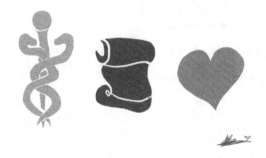

Kevin R Campbell, M.D.

University of North Carolina, USA

World Scientific

NEW JERSEY · LONDON · SINGAPORE · BEIJING · SHANGHAI · HONG KONG · TAIPEI · CHENNAI · TOKYO

Published by

World Scientific Publishing Co. Pte. Ltd.

5 Toh Tuck Link, Singapore 596224

USA office: 27 Warren Street, Suite 401-402, Hackensack, NJ 07601

UK office: 57 Shelton Street, Covent Garden, London WC2H 9HE

Library of Congress Cataloging-in-Publication Data
Campbell, Kevin R., author.
  Losing our way in healthcare : the impact of reform / Kevin R. Campbell.
  p. ; cm.
  Includes bibliographical references and index.
  ISBN 978-9814725446 (hardcover : alk. paper) --
  ISBN 978-9814616812 (pbk. : alk. paper)
  I. Title.
  [DNLM: 1. United States. Patient Protection and Affordable Care Act. 2. Delivery of Health
Care--United States. 3. Health Care Reform--United States. 4. Patient Care--United States.
5. Physician-Patient Relations--United States. W 84 AA1]
  RA412.2
  368.38'200973--dc23
                                    2015029224

British Library Cataloguing-in-Publication Data
A catalogue record for this book is available from the British Library.

Typeset by Stallion Press
Email: enquiries@stallionpress.com

Printed in Singapore

Introduction

As a young biochemistry student at North Carolina State University in Raleigh, NC, I dreamed of providing life saving therapies for patients and grew up knowing I wanted to be a doctor. The promise of the science of medicine seemed limitless and I felt an affinity for the study of biological mechanisms. The intricacies of biological systems and the ability to better understand disease processes and develop new interventions for diseases drew me to deeper study. My parents pushed me to excel in all that I did — academically, athletically and socially. Always supportive and nurturing, I owe much of my success today to my Mom and Dad. This book is dedicated to them and their tireless efforts as parents.

While no one in my family had previously pursued a career in medicine (my dad was an agronomist and my mom a homemaker), I became interested in medicine at an early age. Growing up in the 1980s, I observed Medicine to be a respected and revered profession. Physicians were the pilots of the healthcare industry and worked long hours to provide the best care possible for their patients. It was not uncommon to see local healthcare providers working on the weekends, making house-calls and calling patients at home to check on their progress. Patients always came first and clerical work for most practitioners was at a minimum — mostly dictating notes on patients for charts. Billing was simple and straightforward and coding specialists as well as "meaningful use" criteria did not exist.

Physicians spent years in rigorous training programs and learned how to treat even the most complicated disease. Because of their training, physicians were trusted to make the right decisions and were allowed to assimilate data with gut instinct in order to formulate a treatment plan. There were no "practice algorithms" and there were no pre-authorizations required by insurers. Physicians devoted most, if not all of their time, to patient care — NOT to arguing with insurance companies, battling with unwieldy electronic medical records and utilizing complex (and often ludicrous) coding systems for billing (see ICD 10 and the code for injuries that occur while waterskiing with skis on fire).

During this time in America, regulation and government interference in the daily routine of doctors was unheard of. Physicians provided valuable services to patients and were allowed to develop long-term relationships with patients and their families. These relationships allowed physicians to gain insight into the lives of their patients and prescribe treatments that were most likely to succeed given the social situation in which a particular patient exists. When difficult decisions were needed at the end of life, the physician had a frame of reference with which to make recommendations — the lifelong doctor patient relationship allowed physicians to have a better understanding of an individual patient's priorities and beliefs. Patients were treated fairly and lengthy debates with insurance companies and healthcare executives concerning treatment plans and patient-care were unheard of. Physicians were trusted to make the best decisions for the patient and were good stewards of medical resources. Job satisfaction among physicians in the 1980s was quite high. Medical Schools saw increasing number of applications from young, bright, energetic minds. America's best and brightest competed for the very best spots in the best medical schools from all over the country. Highly sought after residency spots were quickly claimed and those who achieved at the highest levels were rewarded with their choice of training programs. Programs in both primary care as well as specialty services were nearly always filled.

Today, the landscape of medicine is quite different

As medicine has evolved in the US over the last 20 years, many things have changed. With increased political interest in medicine, more regulation was inevitable. Several Presidential campaigns in the last decade have made healthcare a central — and often polarizing issue. The fallout of the politicization of medicine is immense and not at all inconsequential. Autonomy for physicians is much more limited. Government requirements have created reams of electronic paperwork and time with patients has become more compacted and even the most complex patient interactions seem rushed. Rather than spending time bonding with patients during office visits, healthcare providers are scrambling to learn new ICD 10 billing and diagnosis codes, inputting data into Electronic Medical Records and meeting other "meaningful use" requirements. In the midst of all of this change, the patient has become lost — the focus on providing exceptional care has shifted to a focus on survival. Ultimately, the people that healthcare reform is supposed to help — the patients — are going to suffer the most. Those with limited means and limited understanding of complex health issues often require more time with the physician. Under the new system, it is not practical to extend visits and, as a result, many of these patients are marginalized and receive less than optimal care. The physician staring at a computer screen and typing and clicking through a maze of electronic requirements has replaced eye contact, personal touch and genuine empathy. Medical records, electronic charting and billing visits have now become the focus of the physician during the routine visit.

In addition to the enhanced regulatory and government requirements, financial pressures have created a system where physicians must become part of enormous networks — the days of the local family physician working in the town in which he or she was born, treating neighbors and family are nearly over. Doctors are now working for large healthcare systems and this integration has caused referral patterns and care plans to be dictated or mandated by employers, government and algorithms. Access to care for many patients has become a challenge as issues with "networks" remain confusing and many providers are incorrectly listed as in-network when in fact they are not. Growing numbers of physicians are unable to accept many of the Obamacare exchange insurance plans due to low reimbursement rates and this is now creating a significant doctor shortage — ultimately increasing wait times for patients to see a primary care provider.

During my time in Medical School at Wake Forest University, much growth and advancement occurred in medicine. New and exciting treatments and devices were developed regularly and patients saw direct benefit through improved outcomes and improved quality of life. Entrepreneurship and innovation were encouraged and faculty members were provided with protected time for research and development. Academic advances and achievements were recognized and rewarded. Now, academics have been consumed with increasing patient volumes, competition with other hospital systems and the finances of survival in a volatile market. Rather than having more protected time for research and designing new technologies and treatments, many academic physicians are forced to provide more of their time for busy clinical activities, marketing the healthcare system to other referral regions and outreach to smaller outlining communities.

In the United States today, we spend more money per capita on healthcare than any other industrialized nation. Our expenditures dwarf those of our allies and our outcomes are often lacking when we compare ourselves to other developed countries such as the UK and Japan. While spending exorbitant amounts of money on healthcare, we often miss the target and many patients go untreated and do not receive care. Providing care for everyone is a lofty goal and worthy of a national effort in order to achieve universal healthcare coverage. However, as we reform healthcare we MUST preserve the doctor–patient relationship above all else. We MUST allow physicians to continue to practice medicine and make decisions based on experience with the best available data in mind — rather than following a government mandated algorithm. We MUST put the patient FIRST in reform — above politics and personal gain.

Unfortunately, our current reform in the US — the Affordable Care Act — or Obamacare — has missed the mark on each of these points. The ACA has been one of the most politically motivated reforms our country has ever seen. Rather than addressing the problem of a healthcare system that ignores many without insurance coverage, the ACA has become a fight over Presidential legacy and has divided the country like never before. Many Americans see the legislation as a TAX and several highly respected economists see the ACA as nothing more than cost shifting and redistribution of wealth.

Over the last three years, I have written a great deal about the impact of healthcare reform on medicine, politics, healthcare delivery and most importantly — the patient. I have watched the politics of reform erode and destroy one of the most sacred aspects of medicine — the lifelong relationship between doctor and patient. While the goal of providing quality healthcare coverage for all Americans was grand — it has not been achieved. Many that have signed up for the Obamacare exchanges have come from a pool of those who LOST insurance due to the law. We have simply rearranged deck chairs on a sinking healthcare system ship (not too dissimilar from the grand Titanic). I have been saddened to witness many longtime patients leave my care due to lack of access because of changing "network physicians" within the ACA exchanges. I miss hearing about my patient's families, their children (and ultimately their grandchildren). I miss laughing, crying and navigating life's curvy roadways with my longtime patients. I worry about their care and wish that I could do more to provide them with the tools and guidance that they will need in order to manage chronic disease and prevent negative health outcomes. However, as medicine has shifted with the latest reforms, I fear that many patients will not receive the care that they need.

Healthcare reform will have a lasting impact on physicians, patients, medical industry as well as medical research and medical entrepreneurism going forward. In this book, I share my feelings about modern medicine and the impact of reform. This book is an examination of how the ACA has affected EACH stakeholder in the modern American healthcare system. We will carefully explore how the ACA has impacted the physician and how the practice of medicine has changed under the law. We discuss how reform has affected the modern patient and how the patient experience in our healthcare system has been drastically changed. We will explore the politics of reform and how those in Washington have put their own legacy and personal beliefs ahead of the good of the patient. Finally, I will discuss how I believe medicine will be forever changed — how the ACA may reshape the future of medicine. What will medicine look like in 5 years? WHO will be providing care and how will that care be delivered? Ultimately, what will the lasting impact be like?

It is my sincere hope that as a nation we will continue to strive for healthcare reform — reform that is patient centered and actively solves problems. We must put politics aside and create a system that is viable for all stakeholders — patients, physicians as well as politicians and industry partners. We must begin to focus on prevention rather than managing long-term disease — prevention will allow us to get ahead of disease and better prepare our patients and their families for the future. Medicine today does not resemble the medical practice of my youth, nor does it resemble the medicine that was practiced when I was in training at Wake Forest University, The University of Virginia nor during my time as a Fellow at Duke University. Medicine (and our healthcare system in general) has lost its way — we must restore medicine to its grand old days and those who practice medicine must be allowed to put the patient FIRST. While reform is necessary, we must build reform around the doctor–patient relationship — we cannot build the Doctor–Patient relationship around reform if we hope for success.

This book is the result of daily writing — a collection of essays that I have written over the last two years during the development and implementation of the ACA. It is carefully divided into Five Parts, each section dedicated to an examination of a different aspect of the impact of reform on Medicine in the United States. *Part One* examines the impact of reform on the patient and how the patient's role has evolved into what it is today. These essays shed light on what it is that makes medicine effective for patients and how today's patients have changed in response to an evolving healthcare system. In *Part Two*, I examine the way in which the practice of medicine has changed for the physician. I discuss the effects of the added regulatory pressures and declining reimbursement on the ability of the doctor to practice. I also examine the direct relationship of the ACA on physician burnout. *Part Three* is dedicated to the Doctor–Patient relationship. In these essays I discuss how modern technology affects the way in which doctors and patients communicate. In addition, I examine how the ACA has negatively impacted patient choice and has eliminated many long-term doctor patient relationships. Next, in *Part Four*, I discuss the politics of healthcare reform and attempt further to explain why things have evolved in the way that they have. Finally, *Part Five* addresses the future of healthcare in the United States. It is my prediction of the further deterioration of our healthcare system unless we, as both healthcare providers and healthcare consumers, get involved and rally for change.

It is my hope that these essays will provoke thought and stir debate. It is through intelligent dialogue and debate that we will emerge from the land of reform as a better people and a stronger society, that we may stop *Losing Our Way in Healthcare.*

About the Artist

Bek Campbell is a high school student in Raleigh NC. She enjoys visual and performing arts, including drawing, digital art, photography, singing in the school choir, and playing guitar. While leaving her career options open at this point, Bek has a strong interest in film-making.

Bek also enjoys animals and volunteers at a local animal shelter assisting the shelter veterinarian with prepping and caring for cats undergoing surgical procedures. Bek is the proud parent of four rescue animals: three cats and a dog.

Bek is an accomplished artist at an early age — her previous published work includes the cover art for Dr Campbell's first book entitled *Women and Cardiovascular Disease: Addressing Disparities in Care.*

About the Author

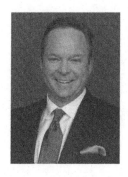

Dr Kevin R. Campbell, MD, FACC is an assistant professor of medicine at the University of North Carolina at Chapel Hill in the division of cardiovascular medicine. Dr Campbell received his undergraduate degree in Biochemistry from North Carolina State University and his medical degree from Wake Forest University. He then completed his residency training in Internal Medicine at the University of Virginia and fellowships in Cardiology and Cardiac Electrophysiology at Duke University.

Dr Campbell is an internationally recognized expert in the prevention of sudden death in women and is the author of *Women and Cardiovascular Disease: Addressing Disparities in Care* (Imperial College Press, London, 2015). Inspired by his wife and daughter, Dr Campbell is passionate about addressing gender disparities in cardiovascular care and speaks to healthcare providers all over the world in order to raise awareness for the treatment of heart disease in women.

In addition to his clinical activities, Dr Campbell is the on-air medical expert for WNCN TV in Raleigh, NC. He is also an on-air contributor for Fox News Channel and the Fox Business Network and appears LIVE on national television in order to provide insight into breaking medical news as well as commentary on healthcare policy. Dr Campbell has been a vocal critic of the Affordable Care Act and has been a highly sought after and respected opinion leader throughout the implementation of the current healthcare law.

Contents

Part One
Reform and the Patient

Introduction

From Hippocrates, we, as physicians, are given one of the most basic premises for the practice of medicine "First Do No Harm". I wonder if politicians in Washington ever apply this premise to the creation of healthcare legislation? The Affordable Care Act (ACA) has forever altered the way in which patients in the US will interact with the healthcare system. No longer does our system put "patients first". Rather, our system now puts bureaucracy and government regulations ahead of patient care.

While noble in its intent to provide affordable healthcare for everyone, the ACA actually has limited access and choice for many Americans. For others, it has forced the cancellation of previous excellent insurance coverage and replaced it with bare bones, higher priced plans. Young professionals, many who are still in school, are being forced to purchase coverage that they simply do not need. Older patients — most who are far beyond their reproductive years — are forced to purchase plans that provide maternity coverage. Why? In order to make a flawed government system work.

Patients in the US have always had the benefit of *choice*. Many patients have developed longstanding relationships with their healthcare providers. Not only are the physicians caregivers but, in many cases, they become part of the patient's extended family.

These relationships facilitate difficult discussions about healthcare decisions and particularly end of life decision-making. Moreover, long-term doctor–patient relationships promote patient engagement. When patients engage in their own healthcare, outcomes improve. With the advent of Obamacare, many patients are finding that their preferred providers or hospital systems are no longer included in their new "networks" of care, as defined by the ACA insurance exchanges. Many notable academic centers of excellence are not accessible due to the fact that the hospital systems have not been able to reach reimbursement agreements with the poorly paying exchange insurers.

Patients are getting longer waits and less access overall, since the advent of the ACA. In this section, we explore ways in which the ACA has negatively impacted the patient experience and how mobile health and the internet have risen to meet the needs of many. We also examine the ways in which care is allocated and who decides where to spend the large sums of healthcare dollars. Ultimately, we hope to inspire patients to clamor for change and work to improve the way in which care is delivered in the next decade.

1

Buyer Beware: How Patients are Negatively Impacted by the Changing Landscape of the Affordable Care Act (ACA)

As the Obamacare machine continues to grind forward, many patients have re-enrolled in a second year of coverage. While most have not had to use their insurance (the young and healthy crowd) others have found their newly minted coverage to be far less than what was promised. High deductibles, and up front out-of-pocket expenses, forced many covered by the exchanges to avoid seeking regular preventative care — prevention was one of the tenets of the Affordable Care Act (ACA) plan. Many have found choices limited and have been forced into healthcare systems that are not their first choice.

Now, as the second year of enrollment (and re-enrollment) has concluded, many of us are concerned about the likelihood of rate hikes and changes in coverage. The Obama administration continues to tout the fact that enrollment numbers remain high and that there have been no substantial increases in premiums. However, this is not necessarily the case. Many exchange insurers have cleverly disguised rate hikes through changes in other aspects of the plans. While some advertise that there are absolutely no significant premium increases, customers who shopped carefully on the exchange site were able to find higher prices for Emergency Room (ER) visits, and higher charges for non-generic drugs. For some plans, this means that rather than paying a $250 co-pay for an ER visit, the customer must pay up to the yearly deductible for the same ER visit before the co-pay rules go into effect. For many, this may be a non-starter. ER visits can be very expensive and can amount to thousands of dollars in just a few hours. Many patients will find themselves having to pay a 3–6 thousand dollar deductible early in the insured year before any of the benefits begin to contribute to reduce individual's out-of-pocket costs. In some plans, the co-payment for a routine physician visit will go down by an average of 20 dollars and many generic drugs will be covered for free. However, specialty visit co-pays will increase and the prices for specialty medications will increase by 40–50%.

In an effort to promote re-enrollment in 2015, the government implemented an automatic re-enrollment system. However, this has left many patients with increasing out-of-pocket costs due to the fact that multiple changes have been made — such as those described above. Many patients were unaware of the need to shop around for re-enrollment and are now increasingly unhappy with their plans. Ultimately, the ACA and its supporters in Washington have placed statistics and politics ahead of the patient. While the delivery of quality care to the patients who need it SHOULD be the goal, it appears that politics remains the top priority. Increasing out-of-pocket costs and higher deductibles — many requiring payment in the first half of the year — are having the opposite effect. One of the central tenets of the ACA is to focus on prevention through promoting regular access to primary care physicians for prevention of chronic disease and its complications. However, instead of promoting an environment where patients are engaged and actively seek preventative care, many are using the insurance simply as a "disaster plan" due to the overwhelming costs. While the Obama administration extols the benefits of healthcare reform in terms of out-of-pocket limits and guaranteed care, the reality is that the way in which the ACA is structured and implemented has actually increased the personal financial burden for many.

What can patients do?

Unfortunately, much of the burden of navigating the new healthcare landscape falls on the patient. The law itself remains a moving target — with changes certain on the horizon. We must remember that insurers are for-profit entities and will ultimately find a way to make a profit — often at the taxpayer and patient's expense. While many have been encouraged by the Obama administration to continue to offer affordable premiums, most have found other ways to improve their revenue streams. Whether it is through juggling co-payments and charges, shifting cost, denying procedure approvals or limiting choice; all of these changes will — in the end — negatively impact patients. As a healthcare provider, my job is to educate patients about behaviors that may improve their overall health. Now with the implementation of the ACA, this responsibility extends to helping my patients manage their insurance choices. While this is not necessarily a traditional role of a physician, it is important that we make sure that our patients continue to have access to the care they need — without incurring a life altering expense.

There are a few things which I think that patients can do to actively advocate for themselves and others:

1. Stay informed: Make sure that you ask questions to your insurer — are there changes to my coverage? How are out-of-pocket expenses handled? Can I see my doctor and my specialist when I want or need to without incurring a penalty or increased cost?
2. Shop around: Just because you have had coverage with a particular company in the past does not mean that you have to remain locked in with them. Make sure you explore all of the

options that are available to you through the exchanges. Carefully question insurance company representatives so that you completely understand policies BEFORE you agree to a contract.

3. Demand transparency: If you are unable to get a clear answer from an insurer about costs and coverage BEFORE you sign up, it is very unlikely that you will get a clear answer once you are a customer. Once you are a customer, make sure that you have a clear idea of the costs involved prior to scheduling a procedure or test. A recent survey sponsored by the Robert Wood Johnson Foundation found that nearly 56% of Americans get out-of-pocket cost information before accessing healthcare services.

As with most things that have occurred with the ACA, it is the patient who ultimately suffers. Insurers continue to profit, as do drug makers and hospital systems and administrators. Physicians have seen reimbursement cut to levels that have forced integration with large hospital systems. Most tragically, however, patients tend to be caught in the middle and have seen their healthcare suffer. Surveys indicate that patients are now inquiring as to cost prior to office visits, tests, and procedures. Many find that they must put off necessary preventative activities and even more opt not to have needed tests and therapeutic procedures due to cost. It is clear that the ACA has missed its mark. While insuring large numbers of Americans is a noble goal, this insurance must also provide value rather than meaningless statistics to be utilized at a White House press briefing. As my research mentors at Duke University taught me during my training — with any data analysis, it remains that garbage in will equal garbage out. WE must find a better way to provide affordable care to our patients. For now, insurers, hospital systems, and politicians are using patients as nothing more than a "Profit Center". As re-enrollment continues through this year and the next, we must make sure that our patients are armed with the old adage — "Buyer Beware".

2

Big Brother is Watching ... And Your Healthcare Privacy Rights May Suffer: More Affordable Care Act Fallout

Data is essential in healthcare delivery and it is often what guides us in improving outcomes. Utilizing data obtained from large populations helps us to decide better what aspects of disease prevention and treatment need more of our attention. These data are important and allow us to evaluate at-risk populations and target our interventions. In the US, participation in surveys is 100% voluntary. The Centers for Disease Control (CDC) obtains most of its data from diagnoses reported by healthcare institutions (there are certain diseases that are mandated by law to be reported). However, with the advent of the Affordable Care Act (ACA), some corporations and businesses have taken the acquisition of data a step too far. The security of personal healthcare data, however, is quite uncertain. In George Orwell's novel *1984*,[1] the author presents a vision of a dystopian society where "Big Brother" watches every move ordinary citizens make in an

---

[1] http://en.wikipedia.org/wiki/Nineteen_Eighty-Four

attempt to maintain order (and advance his own agenda). We have all seen the recent government abuses within the National Security Administration (NSA) and within the Internal Revenue Service (IRS). As the ACA is implemented, I am concerned that Big Brother may already be here and working in the US healthcare system today as well. In medicine, the doctor–patient relationship is sacred — data disclosed for healthcare should be sacred as well.

Although our country has always been grounded upon basic tenets of freedom of choice, right to privacy and other key freedoms, some institutions see Obamacare as a ticket to interfere with the daily lives of American citizens. For instance, as reported in the *New York Times*,[2] Pennsylvania State University attempted to require all employees, including senior faculty, to undergo physical examinations and answer online health questionnaires that contain very personal and very sensitive health information prior to gaining employment and healthcare coverage from the institution. It is obvious that the pressures of the ACA and the need for cost containment motivates and inspires many of these types of mandates. From the business standpoint, the Pennsylvania State University is hoping to reduce risk and liability by modifying at-risk behaviors in its insured employees. However, none of these data will help the faculty do a better job for their employers. So what is the relevance and justification? I am sure that the Pennsylvania State University administration clearly sees this as a way to save healthcare dollars. Saving through prevention and early intervention in at-risk employees makes good sense. However, I am concerned that the next logical step may be to deny or terminate employment based on health risk and potential cost to the system. Where does the rabbit hole end? Is this the beginning of health status discrimination in the workplace?

---

[2] http://www.nytimes.com/2013/09/15/business/on-campus-a-faculty-uprising-over-personal-data.html?ref=health&_r=0

Many senior faculties at Pennsylvania State have refused the mandate based on invasion of privacy, even though the university is planning to levy substantial daily fines for non-responders. Several prominent professors have stated that if they are forced to participate they will simply answer the questionnaires randomly and provide far-fetched ridiculous answers and simply play the conscientious objector. Many other Americans are waiting to see how this pans out and there is concern that this type of activity will begin to spread to other institutions and industries. Labor unions are already beginning to lobby against these mandates and in the case of Pennsylvania State, union employees are exempted. At what point are our private lives and medical histories private? What is the separation between workplace and home? Where do we draw the lines and do we allow others (government and employers) to draw the lines for us?

The spirit of risk reduction and working with employees to improve their health status and live better lives makes good sense. However, there are better ways to accomplish this goal. Health fairs, educational seminars, and free health screenings for cholesterol and high blood pressure make good sense — but all of these activities should be voluntary. Asking highly personal questions such as sexual preference, prior drug or alcohol use and the state of one's marriage should not be a part of a wellness program at work. In the case of the Pennsylvania State questionnaire, there are even questions related to how you get along with others in the workplace — including your boss. These issues are private and should remain that way. In defense of the institution, the development of these wellness programs is not entirely their fault. In fact, the ACA provides a 30% discount for the implementation of a comprehensive wellness program — virtually assuring that every business will "voluntarily" submit to these types of invasion of privacy. Although the university administrators claim that the data is secure and is not available to supervisors and those in the administration, it concerns me greatly that this will not be the case (just ask those Americans who had unlawful wire taps and those who were bullied by the IRS due to their associations with certain political groups). Big Brother is watching ... from your doctor's office, from your bedroom and from your back porch. I am afraid that this particular essay may leave you with far more questions than answers ... maybe we should ask Big Brother.

3

An Apple a Day — Changing Medicine through Technology and Engagement

The practice of medicine and healthcare in general has become an electronic and increasingly mobile interaction. Patients are better informed, more engaged, more connected and have a much greater online presence. In fact, according to Pew Research data,[1] the fastest growing demographic on Twitter are those who are in the 45–65 age bracket. Nearly 50% of all seniors engage online on a daily basis through at least one social media platform and many of these interactions and online engagements occur *via* mobile devices. Almost 75% of all adults go online within hours of attending a visit with their physician in order to gather more information about their particular medical problem. For healthcare providers — and for patients — the internet and mobile technology presents us all with wonderful opportunities to interact, engage, support, and ultimately improve outcomes.

With the increased demands of the Affordable Care Act (ACA) and other government documentation requirements, time spent

---

[1] http://www.pewinternet.org/fact-sheets/social-networking-fact-sheet/

with patients for education and engagement has become even more limited. Patients are reaching out to the internet to garner information about their particular medical condition and bringing much of it to the clinic encounter. Physicians must also use cyberspace as an educational tool in order to make up for lost opportunities during the doctor–patient encounter. As our patients move more confidently into cyberspace and seek information, we as healthcare providers must also have a presence.

New connected devices and medical applications for mobile devices are growing exponentially. The world responded favorably to the latest release of the iPhone 6 and the iOS 8 operating system recently released by Apple. The new device has many interesting features but one in particular caught my eye early on. Apple has created a standard package for all iOS 8 devices that is called the Health Kit.[2] This particular application allows a user to track calories, steps taken (similar to a pedometer), flights of stairs climbed, and other customizable health related data points. These data can be organized into graphs and charts that allow users to track progress and adjust activity levels to achieve particular goals. More impressively, the device will allow other health related applications to organize data in the Health Kit as well. One of the biggest problems with medial applications in the past is that there has never been an easy place to organize, store, collect, and view all of the data together. Moreover, this data is not easily shared with healthcare providers. The Health Kit and Apple may revolutionize this entire process of data collection, retrieval, and sharing — Apple has partnered with a major electronic medical record service known as EPIC electronic medical record.[3] Work is underway to allow the Health Kit data and applications to easily interact with the EPIC medical record. This would allow for easy downloads of health data during a face-to-face encounter with healthcare providers. Currently, most major hospitals and healthcare systems

---

[2] https://www.apple.com/ios/whats-new/health/
[3] http://www.epic.com/

are moving to the EPIC platform. The data collected and down-loaded at one location would subsequently be available to all providers in the system — portability of data allows for better care and less duplication of efforts.

How can we continue to engage?

Much has been written about patient engagement and improved outcomes in the medical literature. While bureaucrats continue to diminish the importance of the doctor–patient relationship and limit our ability to practice the art of medicine, online engagement has begun to thrive. Ironically, while the government would like to create an algorithmic approach to medicine and have automatons as physicians, social media and other online applications have pro-vided physicians and other healthcare workers with new and even more effective ways to engage and educate patients.

Engagement through health applications:
Bridging the doctor–patient gap

I can think of no better way to improve engagement than through the use of real time health applications. These allow patients to receive real time feedback — both good and bad — and respond quickly in order to improve their overall health status. I think that this type of technology will only continue to grow. Apple plans to release the Apple Watch in 2015. I expect that this will also be integrated with Health Kit and allow for the measurement of res-piratory rate, heart rate, body temperature, and other biologic measurements. As these tools continue to develop and applications grow, healthcare providers as well as patients must be receptive to their use. These technologies have the potential to allow clinicians to better assess patients between office visits and provide more directed and timely changes in therapy. Ultimately, I believe these technologies will transform healthcare. As we continue to strug-gle with healthcare cost containment in the era of healthcare reform, the ability to shift care and routine interaction to mobile platforms may very well prove to be a critical piece of the puzzle.

This is an exciting time in medicine as well as in healthcare technology. Moving forward, I look to a day where biologic sensors collect data, relay data to mobile devices and then transmit information seamlessly to healthcare systems. The healthcare providers are alerted to any abnormalities and electronic responses are generated — those patients requiring timely in-person visits can be identified and scheduled, while those that can be handled virtually can be managed quickly and effectively as well. Ultimately, our goal is to manage disease better and improve outcomes. I think that technologies such as the Health Kit and the Apple Watch are giant leaps forward and are just the beginning of a new age of virtual healthcare.

4

Medicine in the Age of Mobile Technology: How Tablets Are Transforming the Patient Encounter

Medicine is becoming mobile. Physicians, nurses, and other healthcare providers must be able to quickly assimilate and react to an overwhelming stream of data. Tablet technologies, such as the Apple iPad, have been incorporated into the workflows of many clinics, emergency rooms, and hospitals. Medical Schools and Residency programs are quickly adapting the technology for teaching. While tablets do present some security challenges, most clinicians who are currently using them tout them as revolutionary and efficient. Moreover, there appears to be many new medical uses for tablet technologies in the pipeline that may forever change the way medicine is practiced.

Tablet utilization: Pros and cons

Many hospitals are now using tablet technology to help physicians and other treatment team members prepare and interact with patients while on the move. With healthcare reform and cost containment strategies, many hospital systems are looking for ways to streamline care and cut costs. Potential advantages of tablet use include the ability to improve workflow on rounds, reduce staffing requirements, and increase productivity and efficiency without compromising patient outcomes. In many centers, physicians are able to "sync" their devices wirelessly or *via* sync stations located throughout the hospital. Rather than moving to a computer terminal to sit down and review labs, consult notes, test results, etc., a team can move through the hallways and discuss these findings *via* an interaction on the iPad. There is virtually no downtime and less staff are required to see patients in an efficient way. When interacting with patients in their room, caregivers can actually show them images and results and discuss findings with them. In fact, a recent study from the University of Sydney showed that secondary review of radiology study images on an iPad was just as good as a standard LCD computer screen. For patients, it improves education and engagement in the care plan when they are able to see an image or test result as they discuss the finding with their providers. When patients have a better understanding of their medical problem and are able to participate in their treatment plans, outcomes improve. Tablet technology helps facilitate this type of engagement.

Some centers are incorporating their electronic medical record (EMR) into the tablet *via* a mobile application and this allows for quicker documentation and immediate record of the day's plan for the patient — available for all team members to access "real time". The EMR mandates put in place by the federal government have become a burden to many facilities and providers — by interfacing with these technologies *via* tablet technology, adoption of EMR and efficiency of documentation may improve.

As with any computerized medical record or medical application, security, and Health Insurance Portability and Accountability Act (HIPPA) regulatory compliance are always a concern. In addition, the small size and mobility of the iPad device makes keeping the devices in the hospital a challenge. Although several major academic medical centers, including Massachusetts General Hospital have begun to incorporate tablet technologies into their practice, many others have not due to the cost of stocking the institution with the relatively expensive devices. Now, many EMR companies, including EPIC (a major EMR player in academic centers) have created secure applications for tablets and other mobile devices that protect privacy and are HIPPA compliant.

Tablet technology: Future applications in medicine?

At this point, we are only seeing the tip of the iceberg when it comes to mobile technology in medicine. Tablets are very powerful, portable, and user friendly. I believe that these devices will become standard issue in medical schools across the country. Rather than spending 1,000 dollars per student on printed materials for a year of medical education, schools such as the Yale University School of Medicine are now issuing iPads to all students and utilizing the iPad for nearly all curriculum related materials. According to the Association of American Medical Colleges (AAMC),[1] tablet technology is being adopted all over the country and is being used to replace reams of learning materials on paper. In a recent survey of medical students published in the *Journal of the American Medical Library Association*,[2] most students utilize electronic-based medical resources at least once a day and over 35% use a variety of mobile devices to access information.

Applications continue to be developed that have important educational roles in medicine-apps for learning electrocardiograms (EKGs), reviewing histology, learning pharmacology, and others are becoming mainstream and will likely be an integral part of medical education going forward. A recently published

---

[1] https://www.aamc.org/newsroom/reporter/december2013/363858/mobile-devices.html

[2] http://www.ncbi.nlm.nih.gov/pmc/articles/PMC3878932/

study in *JAMA: Internal Medicine*[3] evaluated the changes in resident efficiency when using iPad devices for clinical work. In the study, the authors found that the utilization of mobile devices improved workflow and both perceived and actual resident physician efficiency. In fact, orders on post-call patients were placed earlier — before 7 a.m. rounds — likely resulting in improved care and more timely delivery of medications, treatment plans, and orders for diagnostic studies.

For patients, tablet technologies may improve their visit experience and may help reduce medical errors. I can foresee a clinic where patients check-in for their appointment and are given an iPad to fill out forms and answer a wellness screening questionnaire prior to their visit to their primary care doctor. With more "meaningful use" requirements imposed by government bureaucrats, these electronic screening opportunities will allow clinicians to not only meet regulatory requirements but also continue to spend meaningful time with their patients during a visit. In addition, patients can have the opportunity to review imaging with their clinician at their side and actually "see" what the doctor is able to see.

For physicians, the possible applications of tablet technologies are endless. Ultimately, I believe that these mobile technologies will revolutionize medicine and allow for care to be provided to patients who have previously been underserved. Tablet-based electronic patient encounters are on the horizon. As physicians we must ensure that we continue to embrace technology and we must not resist change — medicine remains both a science and an art. We must continue to strive to incorporate BOTH technology and human touch into our patient encounters. Change is coming — we must adapt and embrace these technologies in order to provide our patients with the healthcare and caring that they deserve.

---

[3] http://archinte.jamanetwork.com/article.aspx?articleid=1108771

5

Obamacare Delays and Rearranging Deck Chairs on the Titanic: Old People Can't Surf

Throughout the rollout of the Affordable Care Act (ACA), there have been many delays and several rescheduled deadlines. While many can be traced to political advantage and the timing of elections, there are some delays that have raised eyebrows. During the fall of the initial enrollment year of Obamacare, one particular delay or "accommodation" (as it was termed by the White House) was announced that provided yet another extension for enrollments. The reason given for the delay was that there were concerns voiced by the Obama administration that the "rush" to sign up during the final days may cause delays and result in a website crash. Therefore, it was proclaimed that those who were "trying to sign up" would be given an extension to mid-April to complete the process. Overall there have been more than 20 unilateral changes/delays/exceptions made by the President without Congressional approval or oversight. Exceptions have been provided for businesses and those who serve and work in the Congress BUT the individual mandate remains in place. In the meantime, many who have been counted as "signing up" have no insurance and a large number have not yet paid their premiums. However, the biggest problem with the manipulation of the ACA may actually be the commentary of one of its greatest supporters-Senator Harry Reid.

In early 2014, with the 2014 mid-term elections looming, many of those in Congress who were facing re-election commented on the latest delays in an effort to positively spin the news. As you might expect, those in leadership roles such as Senator Harry Reid have tried to minimize the impact of repeated Obamacare failures and fixes on his part (a desperate attempt to cling to a majority). In an effort to explain the need for the latest delay, Senator Reid has shown his complete lack of connection with the nation. He publicly proclaimed and was quoted in the *Washington Times*[1] as saying that "some [old people] may not be educated about [or understand] the internet". In reality, more seniors than ever before are utilizing the internet in order to maintain medical information. Pew Research Center[2] data indicates that as of 2013, nearly 60% of all Americans in the 50–65 year old age group are actively engaged in internet-based social media. Even more telling is the fact that 50% of those over the age of 65[3] are involved in AT LEAST one internet-based social media outlet. It is clear that the internet and medicine will be intimately connected in the future. Twitter, a popular site for micro-blogging in 140 characters or less has seen a 79% increase in utilization by users in the 50–65 year old age group. When you carefully examine the Senator's comments he is clearly referring to those in the 50–65 year old range — those over 65 will be enrolled in Medicare and have no need to go to the exchanges. The younger populations — such as the millennials — are assumed to be web savvy from birth.

---

[1] http://www.washingtontimes.com/news/2014/mar/26/reid-obamacare-delay-some-folks-not-internet-savvy/

[2] http://www.pewinternet.org/2012/09/15/senior-citizens-and-digital-technology/

[3] http://www.pewinternet.org/2012/06/06/older-adults-and-internet-use/

The delivery of healthcare is already evolving digitally, particularly in the areas of the electronic patient and in mobile health applications. For Senator Reid to make such a statement concerning the inability of older Americans to "understand" the internet not only is insulting but shows a complete lack of connection to and respect for the very people he claims to want to protect. Seniors are more web savvy now and are able to access the web in a variety of ways — there is data from non-biased scientific surveys (such as those conducted last year by Pew) to substantiate my statement. In reality, his comments are a sad attempt to explain the inexplicable — why do the Democrats in Congress continue to hang on to a system that is clearly failing?

The ACA continues to suffer setbacks — most of them at the hands of the President who has dedicated his legacy to its success. The latest delay (or accommodation, as the Obama Administration prefers to call it) is more about the lack of enrollees and less about the ability of older Americans to successfully interact with the internet. Many seniors are surfing on a daily basis. The internet is not the problem with the ACA and healthcare reform — rather it is the legislation that is broken and is badly in need of a fix.

6

The High Cost of Terminal Illness: Big Pharma Cashes in on Hope

As the Affordable Care Act (ACA) enters its second year, issues with our healthcare system continue to expand. We are fortunate in the United States to have access to the best technologies in the world. We also spend more of our GDP on healthcare than any other industrialized nation in the world. Although the ACA does address insurance costs (by passing on high prices to the young and healthy) as well as access (by providing access to care for all Americans even with pre-existing conditions), it does NOT address the escalating cost of drugs and medical devices. I believe that the lack of regulation of the pharmaceutical industry and the prices that they are allowed to set on newly developed drugs is yet another (in the very long list) of major flaws in the legislation.

In the last year, I was troubled by a story in the *Wall Street Journal*,[1] touting the release and FDA approval of a new drug for the treatment of a particular type of aggressive blood cancer known

---

[1] http://online.wsj.com/news/articles/SB1000142405270230328990457919606
4064198886

as mantle cell lymphoma. Mantle cell lymphoma[2] has a very poor prognosis and is very difficult to treat. This new drug has been shown in clinical trials and registries to help treat the disease, but offers no cure. Most patients who start therapy with the drug see 1.5 years of good results, but then no longer respond. For a patient with cancer, time is everything — however the issue with this particular drug is the exorbitant price tag — $120 K annually. According to analysts, the drug could be worth nearly six billion in annual sales for Johnson & Johnson and their drug-making partner Pharmacyclics[3] Inc. The drug is expected to also be approved to treat a common cancer in elderly people known as chronic lympho-cytic leukemia (CLL) and this move will expand its indications to an even more common and larger group of patients.

Doctors who specialize in the treatment of cancers are concerned about the astronomical prices. Certainly, they are excited to have another treatment option (especially a new one that comes in pill form) but they are surprised at the cost of therapy. The new therapy has been shown to be superior to current therapy in clinical trials — however the new drug does not offer a cure. The company supplying the product argues that the cost of the new therapy "is in line with other new drugs for cancer". It seems to me that for pharmaceutical makers the cost is based on what the market will bear — given no limits for cost, they are free to charge whatever they like. It is disturb-ing that those who make potentially life changing (and potentially life extending) therapies profit from the hopelessness and desperation of those suffering with a terminal illness such as rare and advanced can-cers. To me, it is reminiscent of the carpetbaggers[4] after the Civil War.

And cancer drugs are not the only area in which pharma companies are making huge profits. Hepatitis C is a common ail-ment that is transmitted *via* contact with blood or body fluids that

---

[2] Herrmann A, Hoster E, Zwingers T *et al.* (February 2009). Improvement of overall survival in advanced stage mantle cell lymphoma. *J. Clin. Oncol.* 27(4): 511–518. doi:10.1200/JCO.2008.16.8435.

[3] http://quotes.wsj.com/PCYC

[4] http://en.wikipedia.org/wiki/Carpetbagger

are contaminated. It is a costly, chronic disease that can ultimately result in liver failure and death. In the last year, new drugs have been approved that can produce a cure for what has long been thought of as an incurable disease. As with the cancer market, drug makers have offered the drug at a staggering price tag of nearly 1,000 dollars a dose and many treatment regimens cost almost 100 K dollars to complete.

Why is it that physician payments are dictated by bureaucrats — Medicare, Medicaid, CMS, and the insurance companies?
Why is it that hospital reimbursement is dictated by the same?

In the same breath, politicians and others allow pharmaceutical makers to dictate their own terms as to the cost of their product. Are there hands reaching into deep pockets?

With healthcare reform well underway, what is being done to address the cost of drugs? At some point as providers of healthcare, we must step in and advocate for our patients and loudly exclaim ... "ENOUGH".

Many patients struggle to purchase much needed medication while CEOs of pharmaceutical companies continue to receive multi million dollar bonuses each year. Leaders in the pharmaceutical industry suggest that the high price of therapy is a direct result of the capital investment required for research and development (R&D) as well as the costs associated with obtaining FDA approval.

As evidenced by a recent change in the law in the state of Maine, medical consumers are beginning to take matters into their own hands. In landmark legislation, Maine recently legalized the import of prescription drugs from pharmacies outside of the US. There are inherent risks with obtaining prescription drugs from pharmacies outside of the FDA's jurisdiction — there may be impurities and the quantities of the active compound may vary. However, I believe that competition from outside of the US is the only thing that will ultimately bring drug prices in the US back within reach of the average consumer. Big pharma will argue that the cost of R&D requires a high price tag — however; I do not believe that the US consumer must foot the entire bill.

We MUST continue to innovate and produce novel, more effective therapies. It is essential that we support our pharmaceutical industry colleagues in the R&D of new technologies through participating in clinical trials and examination of outcomes data. However, we must stop short of providing big pharma with a blank check to charge whatever they like for newly developed drugs. I am opposed to big government and more regulation in general — but something must be done to control drug cost. Maybe the answer lies in the beauty of the great state of Maine. Maybe if we allow a little competition from the outside, prices may fall and ultimately more patients will have access to potentially life saving drug therapy and hope will not cost a life's savings anymore.

Part Two
Reform and the Physician

Introduction

Today in healthcare physicians have come upon the perfect storm — increasing costs and demand for better access to care have driven reform and limited physician autonomy to levels never seen in medicine. Most of us in medicine entered the field for several common reasons — a love of science, a love of fellow man and an overwhelming desire to apply scientific knowledge to improve the lives of others. In the US, physicians must devote tireless hours to study and work in order to qualify to practice medicine. This time investment amounts to four years of Undergraduate work, four years of medical school and up to 10 years of internships, residencies and fellowships. During these years of training, most physicians are very poorly paid and most subsist on a very modest income. However, the excitement of patient care — the thrill of making a difference — makes the long hours and sleepless nights worth the time investment of nearly 1/3 of our lives in order to be allowed the privilege of practicing medicine. Once in practice, physicians are able to focus their energy on caring for the sick — through direct patient care and through innovations that improve outcomes.

With the advent of reform, the physician's role has begun to change. Rather than "healer" many are finding that they are now forced to accept the role of data entry clerk, coding specialist, documentation expert and government automaton. No longer can healthcare providers focus solely on the patient — administrative duties and electronic documentation requirements overwhelm the clinical time.

Many doctors find themselves coping with burnout and its emotional and professional repercussions. Patient's needs continue to come first but now government regulators have mandated other activities that have begun to erode the sacred nature of the patient encounter. In most offices, a computer screen separates doctor from patient. Rather than eye contact during an encounter, most patients now get to observe the poor typing skills of their physician and rarely are able to really connect on a human level. Many long-time physicians are beginning to wonder if the practice of medicine in its current form under Obamacare is really worth it. Lots of mid-career physicians are beginning to contemplate early retirement and are looking to start new careers in industry and business.

Sadly, it is the patient who ultimately suffers. In this part, we will explore how reform has impacted physicians and medicine in general. We identify the causes of burnout and discuss the symptoms and the ways to identify those at risk. We will also ponder whether or not it is possible to have fulfillment and happiness in medicine today — or is it too late?

7

Reflecting on Medicine and Change: Sailing Rough Seas and Finding Uncharted Waters Ahead

As we closed out on a tumultuous 2014 in healthcare, many physicians looked forward to a better and more stable 2015. For most of us, 2014 was marked by significant changes. Many healthcare providers have seen their jobs and their patient care roles transform completely. Physician autonomy has diminished and regulation and mandated electronic paperwork has more than doubled. Many physicians find that they are spending far less time caring for patients and a greater proportion of their available clinical time is now being spent interfacing with a computer — both at work and at home on personal time. No longer are physicians able to focus solely on the patient — the changes in practice models have now forced many in healthcare to focus on numbers and productivity in order to satisfy the hospital systems in which they are now employed. Job satisfaction rates have fallen sharply among physicians and many have begun to consider second careers. Burnout continues to be a topic of discussion around the water coolers at national academic meetings — irrespective of specialty or practice.

During 2014, we were all been affected by the rollout of the Affordable Care Act (ACA), changes in reimbursement, as well as the implementation of a new billing and coding system (ICD-10). For many of us, it also marked a year of transition to system-wide electronic medical record (EMR) systems such as EPIC and the growing pains associated with such a major upheaval in the way medicine is practiced. Many practices have continued the trend of "integration" with larger healthcare systems in order to remain financially viable. The American College of Cardiology (ACC) estimated that by the end of 2014, nearly 60% of all physician members have integrated with hospital systems and this number was expected to rise even further in 2015 — ultimately sounding the death knell of private practice as we know it. Many are concerned that healthcare will become dominated by only a few large healthcare systems — creating a monopoly. These dominant players may ultimately destroy competition and this will likely result in increasing costs and decreasing care — simple economic principles applied to medicine.

Why have these changes occurred?

Ultimately, I believe that the change to the way in which healthcare is delivered has come about due to three distinct reasons:

1. Declining Reimbursement

Currently reimbursement continues to fall. Multiple government budgetary "fixes" have led to much uncertainty and instability in medical practices (much like seen in any small business with financial and market instability). In addition, the implementation of the ACA has resulted in the expansion of the Medicaid population in the US — now nearly 1 in 5 Americans is covered under a Medicaid plan. Traditionally, Medicaid plans reimburse at levels 45% less than Medicare (which is already much lower than private insurance payments). While the Obama administration did provide a payment incentive for physicians to accept Medicaid, this incentive expired later. Many practices are becoming financially non-viable as overhead costs are rising to more than 60%. As for the ACA, many exchanges have set prices and negotiated contracts with hospital systems — leaving many practices out of network. Both patients and doctors suffer — longtime relationships are severed due to lack of access to particular physicians.

2. Increasing Administrative/Regulatory Demands

With the implementation of the ICD-10 coding system, now physicians are confronted with more than 85,000 codes (previously the number of codes was approximately 15,000). In addition, "meaningful use" mandates for payment have resulted in increasing documentation requirements and even more electronic paperwork. In addition, the implementation of new billing and coding systems has required increasing staff (more overhead) as well as intensive physician training. Sadly, the new coding system that has been mandated by the Federal government includes thousands of absurdities such as a code for an "Orca bite" as well as a code for an "injury suffered while water skiing with skis on fire".

3. EMR Mandates

Federal requirements for the implementation of EMRs and electronic prescribing have resulted in several negative impacts on practices. While in theory, the idea of a universal medical record that is portable and accessible to all providers is a noble goal, the current reality of EMR in the US is troubling. There are several different EMR systems and none of them are standardized — none of them allow for cross-talk and communication. Many small practices cannot afford the upfront expenditures associated with the purchase and implementation of the EMR (often in the hundreds of thousands of dollars). In addition, the EMR has slowed productivity for many providers and resulted in more work that must be taken home to complete — not a good thing for physician morale. Finally, and most importantly, the EMR often serves to separate doctor and patient and hinders the development of a doctor–patient relationship. Rather than focusing on the patient and having a conversation during an office visit, many physicians are glued to a computer screen during the encounter.

So, what is next in 2015 and beyond?

While I have probably painted a bleak picture of medicine in 2014, it is my hope that we are able to move forward in a more positive way in 2015 and the years that follow. I think that there are several very exciting developments that are gaining momentum within medicine and healthcare in general. Innovation and medical entrepreneurship will be critical in moving healthcare forward. Physicians must continue to lobby for the tools and freedoms to provide better patient care experiences for all stakeholders in the healthcare space.

2015 begins with much promise. I am excited to see what we as healthcare professionals will be able to accomplish in the coming years. We must continue to put patients first and strive to provide outstanding care in spite of the obstacles put before us. While 2014 provided challenges, we must rise above the fray and continue to advocate for a better healthcare system in the US today and in the future.

8

Finding Success
and Happiness in Medicine?
Where is the Holy Grail?

Medicine is a very rewarding career. However, recent changes in the healthcare system have made the practice of business much more cumbersome and job satisfaction rates among physicians is at an all time low. Fear over the unknown and how Obamacare may affect our ability to effectively and efficiently care for out-patients going forward has significantly contributed to the general unease in the medical community. Most physicians are highly driven, highly successful individuals. Much of my professional happiness (and I expect other healthcare providers feel the same way) is derived from developing relationships with my patients and achieving excellent clinical outcomes. However, balancing success and happiness in medicine is now more challenging than ever. More time is now devoted to additional government-mandated paperwork, arguing with insurers and managing escalating overhead costs. All told, these tasks begin to take away time normally devoted to patient care.

Recently, I read an article in a business magazine discussing tips for ensuring *BOTH* happiness and success. As I read through the piece, I began to reflect on my own balance of success and happiness — How can these two goals be readily achieved **TOGETHER**? Although primarily directed at the executive/business professional, much of the content is very applicable to medicine. In today's medical landscape, the most successful physicians have embraced the concept of the Physician Executive — developing a business skill-set that allows one to be fastidious with a spreadsheet while also providing exceptional patient care. Now more than ever, it is critical for physicians to think like business people in order to navigate the changes that are being implemented on a daily basis by our government. Although much of our new executive-like tasks certainly take time away from patients, if we are able to find the right balance we can still find happiness and fulfillment in our jobs. As stated in the Inc.com piece, in order to achieve both goals, we must think in unique ways — try to do things differently and find out work which works best for **YOU**.

As a physician, I believe there are six unique ways that one can develop **BOTH** a successful career and enjoy a happy life — believe it or not; they do not have to be mutually exclusive. Here is my take on how each of these suggestions (that were created by Mr. Steve Tobak) can apply to those of us who have made our careers in medicine and healthcare:

1. Develop real relationships: In the end, relationships matter. In medicine, the most important relationship is that with our patients. Understanding patients' feelings, their families and their preferences improves our ability to care for them. Celebrating their successes and their family milestones provides me with great happiness. While the Affordable Care Act (ACA) does not always allow us to continue to bond with longtime patients due to issues with accessibility and networks, we must continue to strive to build these relationships and advocate for our patients and their families.

2. Groom yourself: No, I don't mean comb your hair — Try new things. Engage in other activities as time allows. Make sure that you make time for family outings and that you try skydiving or horseback riding or whatever it is that interests you and give it a whirl. It may change the way you look at your work and your life. Ultimately, exposure to new things can make us all better leaders and provide more opportunities for success at work.

3. Do nothing: Medicine can be incredibly hectic. Running between hospitals and clinics, hustling to see a new consult or dictate another note — all of this "noise" can take away from happiness. Every single day, just take a few minutes to do nothing. Sit quietly and listen to your own thoughts ... meditate. Even a brief respite can make you more effective and ultimately improve your mood.

4. Work for a great company: Whether you own your own practice (a rarity in today's medical world) or work for a university or hospital, make sure you believe in the mission of the organization. Be involved and try to influence policy. If you work in an organization that recognizes and appreciates your efforts, your job satisfaction will improve. If you do not, you may need to consider taking a risk and making a change.

5. Do one thing at a time: This seems like an impossibility for physicians today (guilty as charged). However, if you are able to make a list and prioritize — focus on one or two tasks at a time — you will see the fruits of your labor. Crossing a task off the list gives us a feeling of accomplishment and completion which can add to overall happiness and satisfaction. Trying to chip away at several things at once can often result in no task done well. In medicine, it may be that you spend a half day a week on administrative work — take time to separate yourself from clinical work and catch up on the rest.

6. Be good to yourself: As physicians, we expect nothing but the best out of ourselves — we are often very critical of our own decisions and clinical outcomes. In the current healthcare market (world of Obamacare reform) there is much we cannot control. We must remember to remain centered and remain "in the present" in order to achieve happiness. Although providing perfect care is a noble goal — it is not attainable. Be reasonable with expectations — always provide the very best of yourself to your patients and be satisfied with the fact that you do.

Happiness is critical to a successful and fulfilling career. With sweeping changes in healthcare, many physicians are finding it more difficult to balance both success and happiness. By applying these six unique principles and looking at the "big picture", it is my hope that all of us can continue to serve our patients, continue productive successful careers and remain satisfied and happy throughout our professional and personal lives. If we are able to achieve the right balance then everyone — patients, family, and *YOU* — will ultimately reap the benefits of a long and HAPPY career in healthcare.

9

Obamacare Fuels Burnout: Running for Cover and Finding Nowhere Left to Hide

As the Affordable Care Act (ACA) continues to be implemented, many physicians are beginning to take stock in their own professional and personal lives. The practice of medicine is a privilege but it is also an occupation that can consume nearly all aspects of a physician's life. In the past I have struggled with my own "work-life balance" and I have shared my thoughts on burnout with colleagues and others and have found my writing on the subject to be quite therapeutic. As a healthcare provider, I am absolutely dedicated to my patients and their well being — however, with the new demands that the ACA places on physicians, it may be difficult for many healthcare providers (including myself) to continue to find balance. Loss of balance will ultimately increase physician burnout rates and place an already burdened healthcare system under even greater stress.

Physician burnout rates are currently at all time highs. Symptoms of burnout include emotional exhaustion, feelings of depersonalization and a low sense of personal accomplishment. According to a

2012 publication in the *Archives of Internal Medicine*,[1] physician burnout occurs at much higher rates than other occupations. In fact, *American Medical News*[2] reported that nearly 50% of all physicians suffer from the symptoms of burnout. Decreasing reimbursement, increased workloads and loss of autonomy have fueled much of the current discontent. Now, the ACA promises to add millions of newly insured patients to the system along with more paperwork, restrictions and mandates/benchmarks in order to obtain better reimbursement levels. I am afraid that many providers may be so focused on "checking boxes" for the government that they forget about the patients. Additionally, physicians will be asked to see more patients in less time. As I mentioned earlier, reimbursement levels continue to fall and overhead costs continue to rise. Many private practices have given up their autonomy and "sold out" or integrated with large health systems in order to survive. Now, with the ACA, there are going to be more patients and thus more efficient throughput will be required in physicians' offices. There will be a consistent need for additional staff to manage the increased patient volumes as well as the government-mandated paperwork. However, most practices are finding it financially non-viable to hire additional workers. Ultimately, the shortfalls in staff affect the very people the ACA is established to protect — our patients.

In preparation for the implementation of the ACA, many practitioners have made changes. Many internists are considering giving up their primary care practice in favor of boutique-like practices that focus on hormonal therapies or weight loss. As reported in *Forbes*[3] in January 2013, one in ten physicians are moving into concierge medicine where they charge a limited number of patients an annual fee upfront for 24/7 access to care. One of the basic

---

[1] http://archinte.jamanetwork.com/article.aspx?articleid=1351351
[2] http://www.amednews.com/article/20120903/profession/309039952/2/
[3] http://www.forbes.com/sites/brucejapsen/2013/01/30/1-in-10-doctor-practices-flee-medicare-to-concierge-medicine/

principles of Obamacare is access to care — unfortunately; many primary care physicians are leaving the marketplace just as demand is increasing to an all time high. Physicians that leave traditional practice cite numerous reasons for their exit and many suffer from burnout. Most of us who have chosen a career in medicine do so because of an interest in serving others — selfless behavior throughout one's career. Service to others in our daily practice provides enormous fulfillment and improves job satisfaction. But now, with the ACA in effect, we are no longer able to spend as much time in the service of our patients — we spend more time with government forms, rules and regulations, and are paid little or nothing for the increased administrative duties. The ACA is now one of the primary drivers of healthcare provider burnout and will ultimately result in a physician shortage in the US.

The idea of providing affordable healthcare to all citizens is an important goal. However, haphazard planning and rushed roll-out will most certainly doom the ACA to failure. Unfortunately for all of the uninsured, lawmakers (including our President) have focused more on legacy (and what the history books may say about their time in office) rather than on producing real health-care reform that has a chance to succeed and serve those who need it most. Key components of an effective healthcare system reform include provisions that satisfy the needs of patients, payors/insurers, hospitals (and other centers for care), as well as physicians. Physicians and other healthcare providers are key components to the delivery of quality care — although it appears that our current reform has not accounted for nor planned for physician attrition due to burnout. Failure to provide adequate resources and support for care providers will not only result in quality providers leaving medicine but may also discourage bright young college students from entering the noble profession of medicine in the first place. As many physicians continue to "run for cover" there appears to be nowhere left to hide ...

10

Physicians and Leadership in the Age of Reform: The Power of Applying "I Don't Know" to Medicine

Physicians must be leaders. As healthcare reform continues and the Affordable Care Act (ACA) continues to impact and disrupt relationships between physicians and patients on a daily basis, it is imperative that physicians become increasingly involved in advocating for patient care.

Creating a successful and sustainable healthcare fix is a mammoth task — no one has all the answers. However, saying "I don't know" is not always a negative and may actually be a good first step in the journey toward finding the right answer in the US.

At first blush, we may think that a leader speaking these words may no longer inspire confidence and may lose the support of his or her troops. However, the words "*I Don't Know*" may provide inspiration and motivate teams to perform even better.

As physicians, we are leaders — we lead teams, we lead students and other trainees, and most importantly we lead patients. There are times when we lead and guide patients and families on very challenging journeys through brutal, sometimes devastating diseases. Often, being a good leader is the most important part of our job. With leadership comes many responsibilities and those whom we lead look to us to show confidence as we provide guidance in uncertain times.

As physicians our leadership roles are two-fold:

1. We lead teams of caregivers with a common goal — the best outcome for our patients. Our teams look to us for confident judgments during crisis (such as during a code blue) and guidance when making day to day clinical decisions. Our teams are bright and capable. Our team members are diverse both in training, ability and in education — nurses, physical therapists, pharmacists, and other physicians — all working in concert to achieve clinical success. In healthcare reform, physicians must lead by promoting discussion, advocating for patients and for change and ultimately by engaging those in power in debate.

2. We lead patients and families. We are the experts in a complex field that is foreign to many — we are relied on as guides, as advisors as well as generals on the field of battle. We must inspire confidence and show kindness at all times. Our patients are often frightened and uncertain. We must help them learn, grow, and adapt to changing medical and clinical scenarios.

To lead in this way can be very challenging but is not terribly dissimilar from leading in the business world. We must be prepared — with knowledge of disease and the best available therapies. We must be aware of the strengths and weaknesses of each individual on our medical team (including our own) and we must be able to motivate those in very different roles to band together for common good. We must lead patients and families with compassion — we must understand things from their perspective and apply their needs into the equations we use to make clinical decisions. We must lead both groups with honesty. We must be willing to say "*I Don't Know*" when appropriate.

Then we must harness the power of "*I Don't Know*" in four distinct ways in order to impact change:

1. Creates Possibilities — As a leader, saying "I Don't Know" in medicine, may create an opportunity to bond with patients, families, and team members. Having the courage to articulate your shortcomings as the leader may actually garner more respect and tighten bonds through your honesty.

2. Inspires Engagement — As a leader, saying "I Don't Know" in medicine may provide opportunities for others to take center stage and bring forward ideas that they may have otherwise kept to themselves. It allows others to think more creatively and inspires team members to find "ownership" in working to solve a particular clinical mystery or treatment problem.

3. Avoids Complacency — As a leader, saying "I Don't Know" in medicine provides me with the motivation to learn more and to be better. Not knowing the answer right away drives me to reflect on my particular skill-set and takes stock in what I can do better, both as a leader and as a team member. When the leader works to improve, he often inspires growth among team members as well.

4. Inspires "Fun" During Difficult Times — As a leader, saying "I Don't Know" has a rather positive effect on morale — a culture of "I Don't Know" produces engaged team members and these engaged team members are more productive. Ultimately a more productive medical team results in more positive patient outcomes.

Effective leadership is vital to success in both business and in medicine. The most effective leaders know their own limitations and are not afraid to share that with the team that is inspired to follow them. Courage to say "I Don't Know" may be the difference in discovering the most accurate diagnosis and prescribing the most effective treatment plan for a patient and their family. Be willing to admit when you fall short — as Socrates stated "The only true wisdom is in knowing [what] you don't know".

Moreover, in the era of healthcare reform we must promote conversations with government leaders in order to improve our ability to care for our patients and their families.

11

The High Healthcare Costs of Emergency Department Visits: Stop Pointing Fingers and Begin Offering Solutions

Nothing exemplifies more the complete lack of understanding of the issues surrounding our healthcare system than comments that have been made in the past concerning the use of the Emergency Department (ED) and its associated costs. Many outside of medicine argue that if physicians were more available after hours, the ED visits and subsequent costs could be avoided. While many have written on this subject in the last one year, none have accurately captured the issues involved. While I agree with the premise that ED visits for routine issues are a waste of resources and money, those that suggest that physicians should be available 24/7 and see office patients on holidays and during weekends show a complete lack of understanding of the practice of medicine. In fact, I find these arguments to be down-right insulting to all hard working physicians. Many physicians have spent well over half of their adult lives working for endless hours in training. Many relationships, marriages, and opportunities to bond with children have been sacrificed all in the name of our very noble profession. Advocates for more physician access seem to suggest that if *ONLY* physicians were willing to work during "off hours" and provide cell phone access for patients that the healthcare savings would be enormous. Reality is that if physicians are pushed to do even more and are provided with even less downtime, burnout rates will be even higher than they are now. In fact, I would predict that this type of access requirement would result in a mass exodus of many talented physicians from the profession entirely.

Some misinformed journalists actually write that "many doctors now work 9–5 jobs" — I am certainly not aware of any of my peers who are full time physicians and are working these "bankers' hours". In fact, most doctors in my practice work well beyond the traditional 40-hour work week. As a group practice, we *ALWAYS* have a physician on call for emergencies. However, we do not have office hours in the evenings or on weekends. The cost of overhead for staffing and support makes this type of after hours practice completely unrealistic in the current market. Maybe the solution is for a government-funded healthcare system to train more primary care physicians and have government-run and owned clinics that are staffed in 24/7 shifts. The answer is *NOT* to burden already overworked healthcare providers with more hours, less privacy, and more demands.

However, it is true that ED care on the whole, is costly and inefficient. Some of the blame may be placed on lack of healthcare insurance or lack of personal responsibility for one's own health. Countless patients continue self-destructive behaviors such as smoking, drug use, alcohol use, and other high-risk activities. Some of the blame lies on the "system" with limited access and opportunities for care for some patients (but so far Obamacare has done very little to improve this particular issue).

Some responsibility does in fact lie with the patient — engaged patients who actively participate with their physicians have better outcomes and fewer ED visits. Engagement with a physician does not require having the physician's cell phone on speed dial — it does require personal contact and routine office visits for preventive care and the ongoing treatment of chronic disease.

One obvious aspect that must be added to any discussion of after-hours care must be that of liability issues. Without tort reform, medical malpractice litigation continues unchecked in this country. Many competent physicians have been forced out of practice due to escalating malpractice insurance costs. Many "after hours" messages from physician offices do state to "Call 911 or to Go to the ED" — this is a direct response to the irresponsible litigation that has plagued medical practice in the US today. Physicians are advised by legal counsel to have this type of messaging available in order to protect themselves from lawsuits involving after-hours care. Any real healthcare reform in this country must also include a limit to malpractice awards and the elimination of frivolous lawsuits. These activities also serve to increase the cost of ED care — ED physicians are often forced to practice "defensive medicine" — and order more tests than a physician in another setting might perform for the same clinical scenario in order to avoid litigation.

Certainly, healthcare costs in this country have become nearly unmanageable. I do not claim to have the perfect answer or even a complete solution. The cost of an ED visit is much higher than an office visit with a primary care provider for a routine problem — no one would argue this point. However, the solution is much more complex than Ms Brody will lead us to believe. The answer is NOT to have physicians provide cell phone access 24/7 to patients. The most ideal solution must involve physicians, elected officials, attorneys, and patients all working together to reduce costs and provide better care.

12

The Next Government-Based Healthcare Debacle: Coding for Orca Bites?

Due to the ineptness of the Obamacare team and the debacle that has ensued, the botched rollout of the Affordable Care Act (ACA) has dominated the political and medical headlines since October 2013. However, other healthcare changes are also underway (and have gone virtually unnoticed by the public) that have the potential to further disrupt our ability to treat patients. In fact, the technical and time consuming aspects of these new government-mandated changes may result in even larger scale computer glitches than those seen with the infamous Obamacare website (if you can believe that). In an effort to "better serve" patients and more accurately track disease and document "charges", our government has mandated a new coding system for physicians and other health-care workers.

For decades, the Center for Medicare and Medicaid Services[1] (CMS) has established billing codes for documentation and reimbursement purposes. These codes are created by the World Health Organization (WHO) for the purpose of standardizing diagnoses

[1] http://www.cms.gov/

in order to track diseases throughout the world — it allows for comparative study. However, several governments (such as the US, France, Germany, Canada, and others) have long adopted these codes as a way to standardize billing for medical procedures. These codes have long fallen short of specifically describing what is actually going on with the patient and have led to difficulties in accurately charging for medical services and procedures. In brilliant fashion, there is now a new iteration of the coding system known as ICD-10[2] that will be mandated by the US government going forward. The new coding system, while touted to be more efficient and more user-friendly has become a black hole of government ineptness. Luckily, there are now codes for injuries that occur while skiing on water-skis that are on fire as well as codes for orca bites. As you may imagine, these codes will certainly streamline my ability to treat my patients with these very, very common ailments. Moreover, I (and other healthcare providers) will be spending even more time working on a computer to enter diagnostic codes in order to satisfy hospital systems and government requirements rather than interacting and engaging with patients.

So why is it that our government and its agencies think that their administrators are well qualified to develop codes for medical diagnoses? How is it that bizarre codes for humorous and extremely unlikely scenarios are being included and programmed into the system?

If you ask CMS administrators, they will tell you that these new codes have been adopted by the US government after careful consultation with coding experts, CMS administrators and physician advisors. However, I am not exactly sure which physicians were involved in signing off on codes for "balloon accidents", "spacecraft crash injuries", and "injuries associated with a prolonged stay

---

[2] http://www.cms.gov/Medicare/Coding/ICD10/index.html?redirect=/ICD10

in a weightless environment". The issue at hand is the fact that government is once again working to regulate situations and concepts that they do not understand. Moreover, they mandate changes without adequate input from experts in the field in which they plan to regulate (such as physicians...) While these codes may be better at defining precisely described disease states, they provide little practical utility to the practicing physician. In fact, the ICD-10 system implementation has required that healthcare providers take time away from clinical duties to "train" on the new system. Instead of brushing up on the latest developments in our areas of expertise, we are spending time training as medical coders — ultimately the government believes that it is much more efficient to have physicians and other healthcare providers enter in diagnoses, billing charges, and codes rather than practice clinical medicine.

What are the ramifications of ICD-10 and how it might affect healthcare delivery?

Certainly, if the healthcare.gov website is any indication, I would expect that the technology side of implementation of the new coding system is likely to be plagued with errors and inefficiencies. Imagine developing software that will assist in billing and coding of numerous diagnoses for each patient — including "struck by a macaw" and "bitten by a sea lion" (yes, these actually exist). ICD-10 will increase the number of available codes from 17 K to more than 155 K. From a physician/provider standpoint, the coding process will likely bring efficiency and productivity to a slow crawl as the new codes are phased in. In a survey conducted in 2013, 90% of physicians expressed significant concern over the transition to the new coding system and nearly 75% anticipate a negative impact on their practice (both operationally and financially). Practices and hospital systems will now require new employees (at a cost that ultimately will be passed on to the consumer) who are trained and expert in applying the new codes in order to keep up with government mandates. Over the last year, physicians have been subjected to online courses and training in the new ICD-10 coding system — many leaving the classes more confused than when they began.

Most importantly, however, the new coding requirements will place yet another electronic barrier between doctor and patient. The physician is already burdened with more electronic paperwork — and less time with each patient — and this new coding system will likely serve to further separate doctor and patient. Already, it seems as if we spend more time typing and less time listening and caring for our patients and their families. Where has the "art" of medicine gone? I think that if we were to remove the screen from in between doctor and patient, we may find it again.

Ultimately, physicians will have to change the way in which they document office visits and procedures in order to ensure reimbursement. Altogether, these changes are likely to make an overloaded system even more cumbersome. As we have seen with Obamacare and other government-related policy changes, more work is created, more inefficiencies are exposed — in the end, the patient will suffer. Providers will become overwhelmed by even more government-related paperwork and documentation requirements. More time spent on coding Orca bites means less time in the examination room chatting with a patient. My how medicine has changed …

Part Three
Reform and the
Doctor–Patient Relationship

Introduction

The doctor–patient relationship is a cornerstone for providing exceptional medical care. Lifelong relationships between patient and physician can help facilitate care throughout life and can be essential in dealing with difficult end of life decision making for both patient and family. So much of medicine is based on human interaction and trust — when doctors and patients connect and engage outcomes improve. The development of these bonds does not happen overnight but takes years of interactions and numerous contact points in both the clinic and the hospital over time.

The Affordable Care Act (ACA) has succeeded in negatively impacting this aspect of medicine like no other. When the legislation was rolled out, many patients found that they could no longer see their longtime healthcare provider. Limited choices of insurers through the exchanges and limited "network" physicians forced many patients to choose new physicians and hospital systems. Many providers have been excluded from preferred networks because they refuse to accept the reduced reimbursement rates provided by the ACA Exchange insurance. Many patients are finding themselves waiting for initial appointments with their new physicians due to lack of availability. Many physicians are becoming overwhelmed by the workload imposed by new patient loads, Electronic Medical Record requirements and other government mandated documentation processes. Time with patients has become more limited. Instead of an office visit focusing around a human connection, many patients are finding themselves watching a physician type on a computer. Little time is left for conversation and relationship building. Government interference in the practice of medicine has resulted in a more robotic, algorithmic approach to treating disease. "Meaningful Use" requirements are often irrelevant and inconsequential to patient outcomes.

Ultimately reform has served to separate doctor and patient. If the goals of reform are to provide quality, coherent and connected care to all Americans, the legislation has fallen quite short of expectations. In this section, we discuss the importance of the doctor–patient relationship, how it impacts outcome and how the ACA has limited the ability for physicians to engage in the most important part of our job — connecting with those in need of medical treatment.

13

Limiting Choices
and Destroying Relationships:
Early Consequences
of the Affordable Care Act

Providing healthcare to all is a noble goal. Providing choice, however, is an entirely separate issue. Successful partnerships between doctor and patient are developed over time. These partnerships do not happen easily and mostly, like a long-standing marriage, take a great deal of work. As I have mentioned in previous blogs, when patients are engaged and participate in their care, outcomes are improved. It is easy to see how costs can be lowered through improved outcomes — the focus is shifted to prevention rather than "salvage".

Last year in the *Wall Street Journal*,[1] author Anne Mathews discusses the issues surrounding "choices" in the healthcare marketplaces that began functioning in October 2013. Many insurers began making "deals" with hospitals and physicians — they will be included in their plans as preferred providers if they are willing to settle for pre-negotiated lower reimbursement rates.

---

[1] http://www.wsj.com/articles/SB100014241278873234464045790108004624 78682

Many major healthcare systems such as UCLA in California, Rush and Northwestern in Chicago and Vanderbilt in Tennessee are being excluded as preferred providers in many plans due to the fact that they are unwilling to accept the terms dictated by the insurers. These institutions, and many others like them, employ many of medicine's leaders in patient-care and research. Many patients have developed long-standing relationships with physicians at these institutions and are now forced to make a "choice" — either continue with their preferred provider at an increased out-of-pocket cost or change physicians and start over in their new healthcare plan.

Starting over with a new physician is a lot like divorce. Divorce is not easy — it is fraught with uncertainty and can be emotionally painful. It is difficult to face change when so much time has been invested in building a productive doctor–patient relationship. However, with the implementation of the Affordable Care Act (ACA), patients are now being forced to choose between a doctor they trust and lower insurance premiums. Physicians and hospital systems are being forced to accept payments at whatever level the insurers choose to dictate — irrespective of the cost of the procedure or the staffing and overhead incurred. Once again, the reform of healthcare in the US is doing little to assist the patients who need help the most. Instead of working to build relationships, streamline care and focus on prevention, the ACA has forced "divorce" proceedings on many doctors and their patients. Moreover, the "choice" that is supposedly supplied by the pending healthcare exchange marketplaces has been severely limited. The government cites a lack of time to prepare for the healthcare law rollout — others cite a poorly thought out, complicated and unworkable plan. More than a dozen ACA "deadlines" were missed early-on in implementation and there are changes being made to the law *via* executive memorandum or executive order to this day.

No one argues that the current healthcare system in the US is on life support and badly in need of reform. However, the current ACA plan is not the answer. Based on the basic tenet of coverage for all at affordable prices, the ACA is not living up to its billing. Now, as the law begins its second year, many of the finest academic medical institutions in the country are not going to be accessible to many Americans due to contractual issues with the insurance industry. Ultimately, this will create more of a medical-care divide in the US. Academic teaching hospitals provide cutting edge care and access to new, potentially life-saving technologies before these are available in the mainstream. Those with rare diseases or those with disease processes that have failed other treatments often turn to academic institutions such as Vanderbilt, UCLA and Rush for experimental therapies that may provide hope for a cure. Now, as long as the healthcare exchange plans are able to dictate which physicians and institutions are included in their respective plan, only the wealthy and privately (non-government exchange or marketplace) insured will be able to have an opportunity to participate in ground-breaking and potentially life-saving clinical trials. Ultimately patients will suffer. Ultimately human beings will be denied potential life-saving therapy — all because of limited choice and the coverage "assigned" by insurance companies hoping to limit cost — but at what price?

14

Government Regulation and the Destruction of the Art of Medicine: When Checking Boxes Replaces Care

The practice of medicine has always been more of an art than a science. The great physicians of the past such as Sir William Osler[1] and his contemporaries understood the importance of history and physical exam. These great diagnosticians *talked* to their patients and *listened* intently as the "story" of a particular disease process unfolded before them. This last year, I read an essay by Dr. Bill Frist published in *The Week* magazine.[2] Dr. Frist describes his past experiences as Senate majority leader, as it related to discussions of healthcare reform. I was not surprised to learn that most of the discussions about healthcare policy and reform involved politicians, academics, regulators and lobbyists. The professionals affected most — practicing physicians in the trenches who care for patients every single day — were not even

---

[1] http://en.wikipedia.org/wiki/William_Osler
[2] http://theweek.com/articles/472852/what-doctor-thinks-obamacare

at the table. In the article, Dr. Frist interviews his own internist and asks about how healthcare reform decisions affect his ability to practice medicine.

Several points from the interview stand-out and warrant careful review and comment:

The effect of EMR

A busy internist may care for thousands of patients. Instead of getting to know their patients on a personal level and listening to the "story" unfold in the office visit, physicians are now pecking away at a computer and checking boxes during the allotted 15 minutes. Often, government regulations require that certain questions be asked and documented in the EMR even if they have no relevance to the patient visit. EMR use is important and has many benefits but the computer now can be a barrier between doctor and patient in the exam room. The art of taking a history is to allow the patient to talk and guide discussion. Many times, facts that are critical to accurate diagnosis can be found when the patient is able to tell his "story". When clicking required boxes on an EMR, the physician may unwittingly force the discussion and miss key components. Rather than being allowed to speak freely during the visit, the patient may be simply interrogated by the physician at the hands of the EMR and its boxes that must be checked.

Regulation to reduce waste

Proponents of healthcare reform will argue that regulation will reduce waste and abuse. In fact regulation and increased demands on providers are beginning to have just the opposite effect — more unnecessary paperwork and "box checking" leads to less time actually caring for the patient. With the expansion of healthcare, physicians are asked to care for larger patient loads with less time and with more regulatory red tape. Again, this leads to less time for listening to the "story" each patient so badly needs to tell. Moreover, physician burnout and depression are becoming more commonplace. Increased workload, increased unnecessary and redundant paperwork (even if electronic), decreased reimbursement and ever decreasing quality-time with patients significantly contributes to feelings of diminished satisfaction at work.

Evidence based medicine and quality care measures

As Dr. Frist so clearly points out, checking boxes to meet quality care measures is not what improves care. Compassionate, thoughtful and scientific analysis of a patient's "story" leads to accurate diagnosis and treatment. Treatments based on the best available data produce the best possible outcomes. Physicians must continue to blend art and science in order to make rational treatment plans individualized to each patient. As Dr. Frist mentions this cannot be accomplished by "mindlessly checking boxes". Clinical trials and data, certainly should guide the way in which medicine is practiced. However, in medicine there are no "absolutes". In training, many physicians were taught to never say "never or always" — we must remember that today as well. Data guides practice and evidence guides decision-making, but clinical judgement — not "box checking" makes good physicians great.

The bottom line

Healthcare in the US is in transition. All of us agree that the system does not work well in its current form. Politicians, lobbyists, regulators and academics have shaped the path of reform thus far. Physicians *must* be involved in the planning of the future healthcare system in the US. Although quality of care for our patients is paramount, physicians must be allowed to practice with both the *art* and *science* of medicine. Paperwork, performance measures and "box checking" are beginning to separate patient from physician. We must return the focus to our patients — we must listen to "story" that unfolds in the exam room in order to improve outcomes and impact disease.

15

The Doctor–Patient Relationship on the Brink of Extinction: The Impact of Physician Post Graduate Training

It is unfortunate, but now medicine is "on the clock". We now must not only battle disease, but we must also battle time. Physicians are asked to do more in less time. Innovations such as EMR (which in theory are supposed to increase efficiency) sometimes actually slow clinical practice to a halt. Additionally, ongoing debate exists as to how best to train medical residents and prepare them for the practice of medicine. Technology and Health applications are changing the way in which doctors and patients interact. Training programs have been evaluated multiple times over the last 20 years and sweeping changes have occurred in the way in which the Accreditation Council for Graduate Medical Education (ACGME) regulates the working hours of physicians in training. These changes have a significant impact on the way in which physicians practice once they have completed their residency and fellowship commitments.

Medicine, more than any other profession, is best learned through experiential training. "Hands On" contact with patients and families allows residents to immerse themselves in disease and the continuum of care. Studies from the late 1980s (published in *The New England Journal of Medicine*)[1] suggested that although resident hours were long and arduous, much of their time was spent doing paperwork and tasks such as drawing blood and transporting patients — even in the era of the 100+ hour week for interns only 20% of the work time was spent in direct patient care. In the early 2000s with increasing pressure from politicians and other organizations, the ACGME issued a statement limiting the work hours of house-staff to 80 hours per week. The arguments that led to the limitations in work hours revolved around mistakes and errors during times of sleep deprivation. Citing patient safety and resident "burn-out", advocates for change stressed that care and learning would both improve if rules were put into place to limit consecutive as well as cumulative work hours. However, a recent study in *The Journal of General Internal Medicine*[2] explored the difference in mortality pre- and post-reform. Interestingly, there was no overall change in mortality pre- and post-reform. In fact, when interviewed, residents and attending physicians complained about the dangers of the "patient handoffs". In the old days, the "sign outs" would occur only once a day — in the evening to the on call team. Lists were prepared from every team and a verbal sign-out would occur doctor to doctor and team to team. In the morning, the on-call doctors would discuss the overnight patient events with each team and ensure a proper continuum of care. In the new system with trainees coming and going at different times, there are many opportunities for miscommunication and sometimes important patient care issues get lost in translation. Many times the night call team is not even associated with the particular service they may be covering and may only cover a night or two here and there — resulting in zero continuity of care and no investment in the overall outcome of the patient. More importantly, trainees never truly

---

[1] http://www.nejm.org/doi/pdf/10.1056/NEJM198906223202507
[2] http://link.springer.com/article/10.1007%2Fs11606-013-2401-9

understand the entire course of a disease process as they frequently only see a portion of the span of therapy due to work hour limitations.

Clearly, the current system for training physicians is lacking. Neither pre-reform guidelines nor post-reform guidelines are adequate. This past year in *The New York Times*,[3] author Pauline Chen provided a nice review of the course of reform in medical education. However, near the end of her essay, Dr. Chen makes her most important points — ultimately, by limiting time spent with patients, we are working to eliminate the formation of the doctor–patient relationship. In fact, some data suggests that in addition to a training curriculum for residents most institutions also have a "hidden curriculum"[4] that affects the attitudes of physicians toward their patients once in practice. If the institution is heavy on paperwork and intern "scut work" there is little time for direct patient interaction. These training experiences can shape the way in which the doctor relates to patients throughout his or her career. It is essential that we continue to teach doctors how to be healers. No matter what the working hour limitations may be in the future, we must continue to foster skills for building healthy doctor–patient relationships in our physicians in training. In addition, we must help residents with time management and discover ways to improve the time that they spend in direct patient care while in training. If we do not, we will find that the art of medicine may in fact be lost forever.

---

[3] http://well.blogs.nytimes.com/2013/05/30/for-new-doctors-8-minutes-per-patient/?ref=health
[4] http://harvardmacy.org/Upload/pdf/Hafferty%20article.pdf

16

The Perversity of Medicare Incentives and Reform: Turning People & Patients into 10-Minute Time Slots

As the Affordable Care Act (ACA) continues to impact millions of Americans through its second year of implementation, many things have become clear to both patients and healthcare providers alike — NOTHING is as it seems. While the ACA has provided healthcare to millions of previously uninsured Americans, it has also robbed many patients of their doctors and has forced others into higher premium, lower service plans. Even those with insurance are finding that they have little choice. Many healthcare systems and providers are finding it financially impossible to accept the exchange insurances and many longtime Medicare providers are also opting out.

Why is this happening? Didn't the Obama administration see this coming?

Of course not! In the words of the legendary Nancy Pelosi "We have to pass it to find out what is in it..."

Well, now that we are more than a year into the program, we are all learning exactly what IS in it — more accurately we are finding out what is "NOT" in it ... True *Patient-Centered Care* with a longstanding Doctor–Patient Relationship!

As mentioned numerous times throughout this book, the development of a long term doctor–patient relationship is critical to the successful management of chronic disease. We see time and time again from large studies focused on patient engagement in conditions such as hypertension and diabetes that when patients are engaged in their own healthcare, outcomes improve. Patient engagement does not happen overnight — it requires work and an investment of time and energy by BOTH doctor and patient. A key component to engagement is the development of trust between doctor and patient. The development of meaningful trust and a productive doctor–patient relationship is a process that is cultivated and managed over TIME. Doctors and patients must be given the opportunity to bond and connect. However, this luxury is now more commonly in short supply.

Physicians have found the ACA to provide significantly lower reimbursements and Medicare continues to make further payment cuts. If you carefully look at the way incentives within the Medicare code are structured, you begin to see that they are NOT in the best interest of EITHER the patient or the physician. For example, a 10- minute office visit is reimbursed in some areas at $50 and a 40- minute visit is reimbursed at $140 — with the reimbursement for each block of time reduced in a nonlinear way. While physicians would much rather spend more time with each patient — working on prevention and goal setting AND actually developing lasting relationships — Medicare and other government based healthcare plans seem to incentivize the opposite. In order to remain financially viable, a practice must see more people in less time — reimbursement favors larger numbers of short visits rather than fewer, extended, more productive visits. Overall healthcare costs are not impacted because we are not able to spend needed time on preventative efforts. Patients are not engaged and outcomes suffer.

Say what you mean and mean what you say!

Medicare bureaucrats and federal healthcare regulators say that they would like physicians to *emphasize* patient education, patient engagement and patient inclusion in decision making yet they are unwilling to compensate doctors for the time these activities require. In fact, the current system pushes the opposite — mass production of patient visits with limited time for questions and lifestyle modification discussions. Healthcare providers are actually negatively impacted when they spend more time with patients — often to the point of not being able to remain open and independent without "selling out" to large healthcare systems in order to meet the demands of business overhead. How can we reconcile this with the rhetoric coming from the White House?

Most disturbing, however, is the negative impacts these regulations and perverse incentives have on patients and overall patient care. Patients depend on doctors to advise them and to help them make healthcare choices. While patients are much better informed now — mainly due to the availability of information on the internet — they still need to have quality, non-rushed, personal interaction with a physician. Many patients feel lost and abandoned when they realize that the time they now get with their doctor is significantly limited or eliminated altogether (as many physicians substitute allied health professionals for themselves during routine office visits). While Nurse Practitioners and Physician Assistants are critical to delivering care, they should not serve as a substitute for a visit with the Physician. These healthcare professionals are very good at bonding with patients and delivering routine care BUT in order to maintain a healthy doctor–patient relationship, the physician must find time to interact face-to-face with the patient — even if it means lower reimbursement.

Ultimately time will tell. It is my hope that we can somehow reverse the course of the Obamacare disaster in the years to come. We must find a way to insure and care for all Americans in a way that also allows Doctors to be Healers rather than government automatons. The practice of medicine remains a privilege — we must all work to ensure that the sanctity of the doctor–patient relationship is preserved in the future. We must reform both the ACA as well as the often perverse and misguided, misplaced and misinformed Medicare code in order to allow physicians to provide what is most important to patients and families alike — TIME and PERSONAL ATTENTION. Only then will we have a system that actually works.

17

Sharing Bad News or Keeping Secrets: How Physician Communication Impacts Patients and Families

Doctors and patients bond over time. Information exchange, education and sharing of expertise are critical activities that add to the effective practice of medicine. Delivering bad news is unfortunately an unpleasant part of a physician's job. Honesty, empathy and clear communication are essential to delivering news to patients and their families — even when the news is unpleasant or unexpected. While communication is an integral part of the practice of medicine, not all healthcare providers are able to relay information or test results in a way that is easily digested and processed by patients. Some physicians may avoid delivering bad news altogether — often keeping patients in the dark. While a paternalistic approach to medicine was accepted as the *status quo* for physician behavior in the 1950s, patients now expect to play a more active role in their own care. Patients have a right to demand data and understand *why* their healthcare providers make particular diagnostic and treatment decisions.

Recently, a disturbing report[1] indicated that in a database of Medicare patients who were newly diagnosed with Alzheimer's disease, only 45% were informed of their diagnosis by their physician. While shocking, these statistics mirror the way in which cancer diagnosis were handled in the 1950s with many doctors choosing not to tell patients about a devastating health problem. With the advent of better cancer therapies and improved outcomes, now we see that nearly 95% of all patients are informed of their cancer diagnosis by their physician.

How can this be? Why would a physician NOT tell a patient about a potentially life changing diagnosis?

I think that there are many reasons for this finding in Alzheimer's disease and that we must address these issues in order to provide ethical and timely care to our patients.

1. **Time constraints:** electronic documentation requirements and non-clinical duties allow for less time spent with each patient. In order to deliver bad news such as a terminal diagnosis, a responsible physician must not only spend time carefully delivering a clear message but must also be available to handle the reaction and questions that will inevitably follow. Many physicians may avoid discussing difficult issues due to the lack of time available to help the patient and family process a diagnosis. We must create ways to diminish the administrative burden on physicians and free them up to do more of what they do best — care for patients. More reasonable and meaningful documentation requirements must be brought forward. Currently, many physicians spend far more time typing on a computer rather than interacting in a meaningful way with patients during their office visits. Eye contact, human interaction and empathy are becoming more of a

---

[1]http://www.npr.org/blogs/health/2015/03/24/394927484/many-doctors-who-diagnose-alzheimers-fail-to-tell-the-patient

rarity in the exam room. This certainly limits the effective delivery of bad (or good) news to patients. Priority MUST be placed on actual care rather than the computer mandated documentation of said "care".

2. **Dwindling long term doctor–patient relationships:** networks of hospitals, providers and healthcare systems have significantly disrupted traditional referral patterns and long term care plans. Many patients who have been enrolled in the ACA exchanges are now being told that they cannot see their previous providers. Many physicians (even in states such as California) are opting out of the Obamacare insurances due to extremely low reimbursement rates. Patients may be diagnosed with a significant life changing illness such as Alzheimer's disease early in their relationship with a brand new healthcare provider. When a new physician provides a patient with bad news — of a life-changing diagnosis that will severely limit their life expectancy as well as quality of life — patients often have difficulty interpreting these results. Healthcare providers that have no relationship with a patient or family are at an extreme disadvantage when delivering negative healthcare news. Long-term doctor–patient relationships allow physicians to have a better understanding of the patient, their values and their family dynamics. This "insider knowledge" can help facilitate difficult discussions in the exam room.

3. **Lack of effective therapies to treat the disease:** No physician likes to deliver bad news. No doctor wants to admit "defeat" at the hands of disease. It is often the case where some healthcare providers will not disclose some aspects of a diagnosis if there are no effective treatments. I firmly disagree with this practice of withholding relevant information as I believe that every patient has the right to know what they may be facing — many will make significant life choices if they know they have a progressively debilitating illness such as Alzheimer's disease. In the 1950s, many patients were not told about terminal cancer diagnoses due

to the lack of effective treatments. However, medicine is no longer paternalistic — we must engage and involve our patients in every decision.

4. **Lack of physician communication education:** As medical students we are often overwhelmed with facts to memorize and little attention is given to teaching students how to effectively interact with patients as well as colleagues. Mock interviews with post-interview feedback should be a part of pre-clinical training for physicians. We must incorporate lectures on grief and the grieving process into the first year of medical school. Making connections with patients must be a priority for physicians in the future — we must equip trainees with the tools they need for success. Leaders distinguish themselves by the way in which they share bad news. According to *Forbes* magazine, the critical components of sharing bad news include — accuracy of communication, taking responsibility for the situation, listening, and telling people what you will do next.

What's next?

As with most things in medicine, change often occurs "around" healthcare providers without direct physician input. Physicians are appropriately focused on providing excellent care and connecting with patients while politicians and economists craft the future of medicine. The issues with lack of communication of negative findings with patients MUST be addressed. Patients have a right to their own data and have a right to know both significant and insignificant findings. In order to avoid situations where patients are not fully informed about their medical condition, we must continue to remain focused on the patient — even if it means that other clerical obligations are left unattended.

18

Attending a Funeral: Mourning the Loss of a Friend and Learning More About the Art of Medicine

One of the best things about the practice of medicine is the ability to develop long term relationships with patients and their families. As physicians, we have the unique privilege of meeting and interacting with thousands of people throughout our careers. Every once in a while, there are certain people who really make a lasting impact and forever change us as caregivers and as human beings. Ed was one of those patients.

This week, I said goodbye to one of my longtime patients and dearest friends. Ed, a Korean war veteran, was an amazing man. He was a dedicated father, a devoted spouse and lived a life that was an example of faith and service to others. I met Ed through his daughter years ago. He had moved locally to live near his children and needed a new cardiologist. Fortunately for me, his daughter asked me to take him on as a patient.

Ed had an ischemic cardiomyopathy and suffered from complications of congestive heart failure (CHF). He was fairly well compensated on medical therapy but continued to have worsening

CHF. During the course of his illness, we eventually implanted a Biventricular ICD and his symptoms improved significantly. As with most patients with CHF, over the years, he began to have more frequent hospitalizations for CHF exacerbations.

Through it all, Ed was always cheerful and never complained — in fact it was sometimes difficult to monitor his symptoms due to his demeanor. Ed always put others before himself. His wife, suffering from her own chronic illness, was the focus of his final days. He loved her deeply and wanted to be sure that she was comfortable and well cared for. Because of my relationship with Ed and his family, I have been made a better cardiologist, and most importantly, a better man.

Men like Ed are few and far between — I was honored to care for him. My professional role as his cardiologist is what provided me with the fortunate opportunity to be a part of his life and develop a relationship with him and his wonderful family. As I have said many times before, medicine is best practiced when relationships and tight bonds are formed between doctor and patient. As I left the chapel where the Catholic Mass celebrating Ed's life was held, I could only wonder if I would ever have the chance to meet another "Ed". Healthcare in the US has become more fragmented than ever and care is no longer contiguous in many cases. Many patients are experiencing access issues and are being told that they can no longer see their longtime physicians because of "network" issues or insurance coverage rules. Doctors are forced to spend more time typing and glaring at computer screens and less time actually getting to know the "people" behind the diseases they treat. Connections like I had with Ed are harder to form and personal bonds are less likely to occur in the current environment. I fear that medicine is becoming more about the "system" and managing regulation than it is about listening and caring for those who suffer from disease.

Ed taught me many things during the time that I cared for him. He taught me humility, kindness and selflessness — I have never met anyone quite like him. Most importantly, he taught me the value of relationships and TIME. Even in death, he inspires me to be more to each of my patients — inspite of increasing government demands on both my time and talents. Ed never stopped caring for others — he never wavered in his commitments to his God, his wife and his children. It is my hope that I can stand firm and continue to fight for my patients and their right to receive exceptional care. While I continue to actively speak out against the Affordable Care Act and the regulation of medicine that separate doctor from patient, I must do so in a way that is constructive and advocates for the patient rather than for the doctor. That is how Ed would see it — of that I am sure.

Part Four
The Politics of Reform

Introduction

Politicians have now assumed control of medicine and political agendas have become paramount to patient outcomes. In the last decade, we have seen physicians lose autonomy and medical care has begun to be dictated by those in Washington. Meanwhile, administrators in healthcare and CEOs of large healthcare companies and hospital systems have increased by nearly 3,000%. Physicians have been relegated to punching time clocks and answering to men and women in suits.

The Affordable Care Act (ACA) promised so much to so many but has delivered so little to so few. Presidential legacies have taken priority over passing legislation that actually works and meets the needs of an aging American population. When physicians met the ACA with skepticism, the government promised that once implemented the ACA will provide an optimal healthcare experience for all — patient, doctor and insurers. However, after more than two years of Obamacare all parties have realized that the legislation has been nothing more than a "bait and switch" on the part of the Obama administration.

Choice of provider, healthcare system and setting has been limited and removed from the patients' hand. While costs remain constant, care has become more fragmented. Politicians in Washington continue to stick their collective heads in the ground and refuse to compromise in any meaningful way in order to "fix" the disaster that is the ACA. Longstanding doctor–patient relationships are beginning to find interruption due to changes in "preferred providers" and access for many newly insured patients is limited.

It is clear that the ultimate goal of the Obama administration was to simply pass legislation in order to go down in history as the President who reformed healthcare — no credence was given as to whether or not the reform legislation was effective and improved the lives of the average American. Thus far, it has become another unwieldy, ineffective and wasteful government program.

In this section, we explore how the politics in Washington have shaped healthcare reform and how little legislators actually knew about the bill when passed. Through these essays, I explore how ultimately patients and outcomes will suffer. Furthermore, I will describe how our healthcare system — once focused on doctor and patient — is now centered around big business, big government and big profits for hospitals. Ultimately, it is my hope that this book will be a rallying cry for patients and physicians to demand better healthcare and to demand that politicians remove themselves — and their egos — from the practice of medicine.

19

Sex, Lies and Healthcare Reform: The Current (Sad) State of the (Un) Affordable Healthcare Act

In the first year of the Affordable Care Act (ACA) many changes in leadership occurred as the White House began to duck for cover during the shaky rollout. Ultimately, the US House of Representatives finally got the opportunity to question the first leader of the ACA program — Secretary Kathleen Sebelius — and examine the debacle that is the ACA. Unfortunately, the Secretary of Health and Human Services spent most of the three hour session skirting around the issues and tossing blame to other government agency bureaucrats, government contractors and of course the GOP (Grand Old Party). When repeatedly pressed, she did in fact admit responsibility for the failed rollout but stopped short of admitting that the ultimate responsibility falls upon the Commander-in-Chief, President Barack Obama. Like any good soldier in a politically appointed job, she protected her boss from the fallout of the *TRUTH*. However, in spite of the Secretary's claims of ignorance during her testimony, lawmakers on the House committee as well as the American people were able to begin to better understand why the ACA has been such a disaster:

1. A complete lack of leadership on the part of the President and his appointees.
2. A complete lack of understanding of the law by the very people who drafted and now champion the legislation.
3. A complete lack of understanding of the process of healthcare delivery in the US today.

For example, numerous provisions have already been delayed and many more are likely to be postponed in the future. The mandates on some businesses, the out-of-pocket expense caps, and now the individual mandate — just to name a few. Throughout the process there have been many misleading statements made by the President and his political colleagues both in the White House and on Capitol Hill. No less than six different statements were made by Mr. Obama forcefully claiming in 2009 while addressing the American Medical Association:

> "If you like your doctor, you will be able to keep your doctor, period. If you like your health care plan, you'll be able to keep your health care plan, period. No one will take it away, no matter what."

Obviously the hundreds of thousands of insured that are now being dropped by their insurance plans and forced into the exchanges are proof that these statements are in fact not true. In addition, there is mounting evidence that the White House as well as Secretary Sebelius knew about these issues with potential coverage loss for quite some time. An IRS document[1] from 2010 (during the time in which the President was making such bold statements about coverage) suggested that this may in fact not be the case. This document clearly states that an estimated 40–60%

---

[1] http://www.irs.gov/irb/2010-29_IRB/ar08.html

of individual policyholders would be dropped from their plans due to the ACA. An article in the *Washington Post*[2] awarded the administration with "Four Pinocchios"[3] for making untrue claims about his cherished ACA.

We are a nation built on certain guaranteed freedoms — in particular freedom of choice, freedom of religion and freedom of speech — we are slowly losing our way in the healthcare debate. Those with particularly stringent religious beliefs concerning pre-marital sex and birth control practices are now forced to purchase products that supply contraception. The Catholic Church — whose believers practice natural family planning — are being forced to provide their employees with funding for birth control. Our government has clearly overstepped its bounds. Those who are healthy and have little need of expensive insurance policies are now forced to pay for benefits they may not really need. The entire success of the ACA system requires that those who do not need medical care pay for those who do — a unique system for transferring wealth.

Ultimately, costs will continue to rise. As evidenced by a report filed by Sebelius's very own Health and Human Services (HHS)[4] in September 2013, most will see a significant premium increase. The average male in the US today who enters the exchange will see a 99% increase — the average female will see a 67% increase. In some states such as North Carolina where I reside, the average man will pay a 350% increase in premium. Rather than closing the wealth gap in the US, the ACA will actually result in the development of two divergent classes of Americans with respect to healthcare — those with wealth will be able to pay out-of-pocket for concierge medicine — they will have access to whatever they need, whenever they need it as long as they can continue to pay.

---

[2]http://www.washingtonpost.com/blogs/fact-checker/wp/2013/10/30/obamas-pledge-that-no-one-will-take-away-your-health-plan/?hpid=z1
[3]http://www.washingtonpost.com/blogs/fact-checker/about-the-fact-checker/
[4]http://aspe.hhs.gov/health/reports/2013/MarketplacePremiums/ib_marketplace_premiums.cfm

The rest of America will be lumped into the dysfunctional and bureaucratic Obamacare system.

I am sadly disappointed by my government — those in charge have slowly chipped away at my noble profession — medicine is in jeopardy of no longer being a form of art soon medical care will be an automated system carried out by a group of mindless lemmings. The doctor–patient relationship which has been the core of good medical care is in danger of extinction. I am a firm supporter of providing healthcare to those who cannot afford it — just not at the cost of freedom. I can only hope that those in power in Washington will respect the basic tenets of our democracy and, most importantly, put legacy and ego aside and help us do what we do best as doctors — put patients first.

20

Obama's Latest Bait and Switch for Docs: Medicaid Payments to be Cut by 40%

As we enter year two of the Affordable Care Act (ACA), we have seen many issues arise during implementation. Through both executive order and executive memorandum, President Obama has unilaterally changed the law more than 100 times in order to advance his own political agenda. When it became important to publicize enrollment and increase coverage of the uninsured, the President and the ACA provided for an increased payment scale for patients with Medicaid. With the rapid increase of Medicaid insured patients due to the implementation of the ACA, the administration utilized the increased payments as an incentive to attract more physicians to participate in Medicaid programs. According to the *New York Times*,[1] the ACA has resulted in the largest increase in Medicaid covered patients in history — now nearly 20% of all Americans are covered under this plan. Attracting physicians to cover Medicare patients has been critical in order to

[1]http://www.nytimes.com/2014/12/28/us/obamacare-medicaid-fee-increases-expiring.html?hpw&rref=health&action=click&pgtype=Homepage&module=well-region&region=bottom-well&WT.nav=bottom-well

meet the demand for access to care and to adequately cover the newly insured. Now, unless changes are made soon, Medicaid reimbursements will be cut once again leaving many physicians to wonder if they can continue to treat the increasing numbers of Americans covered through these programs.

Traditionally, Medicaid has reimbursed physicians at rates significantly lower than Medicare making practices with large numbers of Medicaid patients financially non-viable. As the ACA was rolled out, a provision was made for significantly better Medicaid payment rates to physicians in order to help provide larger networks of care for the newly insured. Now, there looms an automatic payment rate cut of nearly 43% for Medicaid payments to primary care physicians — many of these are the same physicians who agreed to expand Medicaid within their practices in order to meet demand. According to *Forbes*,[2] traditional Medicaid reimbursement averages just 61% of Medicare reimbursement rates (which is often significantly lower than private insurance rates). In addition, many Medicaid patients require a disproportionate amount of time and resources from the office — doctors are caught between a "rock and a hard place" — between a moral obligation to treat these patients and a desire to avoid financial ruin. These patients tend to be sicker, have multiple medical problems and have suffered from a longtime lack of preventive care.

Finances are not the only piece of the Medicaid puzzle. Government regulation and paperwork and processing often delays payments to physicians and impacts their ability to run a financially sound business. Interestingly, a study from 2013 published in *Health Affairs*[3] suggested that while physicians welcomed an increase in reimbursement rates as incentive to treat Medicaid patients that quickened payment times, reduced paperwork and

---

[2]http://www.forbes.com/sites/peterubel/2013/11/07/why-many-physicians-are-reluctant-to-see-medicaid-patients/
[3]http://content.healthaffairs.org/content/32/9/1560.abstract

simplified administrative processes would also need to be a part of any type of reform (of course, none of these items were included in the incentive package).

Many primary care physicians stepped up to answer the call for increasing coverage of Medicare patients when the ACA was initially rolled out. Now, these same physicians are contemplating the need to drop these patients from their clinics with the pending change in reimbursement. As mentioned above, in addition to lower reimbursement rates, the Medicaid program requires an enormous amount of administrative work in order to file claims and these claims are often paid very late — those running a small practice are forced to work more for less pay and often have to make difficult budgetary decisions in order to payroll for their staff each week. While the administration touts the swelling numbers of Medicaid covered patients — nearly 68 million currently — I suspect access to quality care will soon become an issue. Just as with every other manipulation of the ACA over the last two years, legacy and political agendas have taken precedent over what really should matter — providing quality medical care AND prompt, easy access to care for the formerly uninsured. In an effort to tout swelling numbers of "covered" Americans, the Obama administration has failed to anticipate the impact of short term financial incentives for primary care physicians to accept increasing numbers of Medicare patients. Even in states such as California, officials are bracing for a large number of physicians who have announced that they will likely drop out of Medicaid plans if the planned cuts are implemented as scheduled.

It is time for the Obama administration to stop playing political games with our healthcare. If the mission of the ACA is to provide affordable quality healthcare for all Americans, then we need to ensure that there are quality, dedicated physicians available to provide that care. The Medicaid "bait and switch" is just one example of our President's shortsightedness and lack of connection to those dedicated physicians who work tirelessly to ensure that ALL patients have access to care (regardless of insurance type). It is my hope that the new Congress will engage with the physician community and find real solutions to the US healthcare crisis — and no longer allow the President to place his perceived legacy over the healthcare of those Americans who are in need.

21

Unsustainability: Obamacare, Medicaid Expansion and the Destruction of the "Art" of Medicine

During this last year, I have reflected on the last year and the many good things that we have all been blessed with in healthcare. I have the opportunity to serve patients and their families every single day. I have the privilege of making a difference in the lives of others. However, as I reflect, I am greatly troubled by what looms in the year ahead for physicians and their patients.

As Obamacare continues into its second year, other programs such as Medicaid are expanding as well. Already overwhelmed US healthcare systems continue to be flooded with new patients. Experts argue that the Medicaid expansion will allow for "timely access" for all new patients. However, once again, the Obama administration has failed to look at one of the core problems with expansion — who the heck is going to treat all of the new patients? The current expansion of Medicaid (in concert with the Obamacare mandate) is likely to result in long wait times for primary care office visits, limited subspecialist access to those with the worst insurance (Medicaid) and ultimately poorer outcomes for patients.

Some experts predict a significant shortage of physicians (both primary care and specialists) as we race to meet the flood of newly insured patients. During the design of the expansion of Medicaid, no one with actual experience in caring for patients has seriously considered how the care they plan to provide will be delivered. Traditionally, Medicaid reimbursement rates are significantly lower and the payment process is filled with bureaucracy, paperwork and red tape. As discussed in the *New York Times*[1] in the last year, the Medicaid expansion in California is underway. Over 9 million people will enroll in the Medicaid programs expanding all across the US very soon. But many doctors will be unable to accept Medicaid patients due to the low rates of payment included with the program — for example — in California where we have one of the largest Medicaid populations in the US, only 57% of physicians will accept Medicaid. Many subspecialists will not — financially it is not feasible to pay increasing overhead costs, increasing malpractice premiums and receive reimbursement rates that are well under even traditional Medicare rates. In fact, many physicians in California who have traditionally accepted Medicaid patients will no longer be able to take on new ones. In response, the government has issued "incentives" to persuade physicians to accept new Medicaid patients. These incentives include "higher" reimbursement rates for two years (then the rates revert back to the mean at that time) — what they do not tell you is that the increased rates are still below standard CMS Medicare reimbursement.

How is this changing the landscape of healthcare delivery?

Clearly, we must provide care to all Americans. We must, however, do it in a way that makes good financial sense. The practice of cutting rates for physicians and expecting them to continue to work 60+hour weeks, sacrifice family-time and meet increasing demands

[1] http://www.nytimes.com/2013/11/29/us/lack-of-doctors-may-worsen-as-millions-join-medicaid-rolls.html?pagewanted=1&ref=health

of electronic documentation and higher patient loads is unsustainable. As physicians, we are part of a noble profession and we all care deeply for our patients. Our passion is to help others battle disease. We consider much of what we do to be **SERVICE** and the rewards for service to others are immeasurable. However, physicians sacrifice a great deal of time to become experts in their respective specialties. Some of us have endured as much as 10 years of post MD graduate training with low pay and long hours. Many have mountains of school loans and debt to repay.

From a business perspective, many physicians are finding shelter under the cover of large healthcare systems and hospitals — both private and university based. The private group or traditional private practice is becoming extinct. Competition is beginning to dwindle in many markets as hospital systems gobble up other institutions and other groups that once competed for patients — essentially forming monopolies of healthcare delivery. Add to the realignment of groups and hospitals the newly formed Exchanges that have limited choice and healthcare prices are no longer subject to free market competition.

What are the options? Healthcare is a business, right? Or is it simply another government program?

I certainly do not claim to have all the answers. However, I do recognize that the course that the Obama administration has set upon is unsustainable. We will soon be facing a crisis of physician shortages throughout the US. Medicine, although a noble and honorable profession, is no longer an attractive option for many of our brightest young minds. Of the physicians (like myself) that continue to practice and care for our patients with passion, burnout is common. If we continue to limit reimbursement and increase workload, physician burnout will continue to rise at levels much higher than in the past.

Maybe the answer is for the government to create a federally run health service. In this model, the government selects prospective medical students and funds their medical training — pays for medical school and living expenses during internship, residency and fellowship training. Once training is completed, the young physicians are then obligated to practice in a government owned hospital or clinic for a number of years (commensurate with the number of years that they benefited from government support). The government would control their salary, their work hours and their practice location. All patients who are signed up for Medicaid are then assigned a clinic and a physician from which they will receive their care. Those who choose not to participate in government clinics will most likely be a part of "boutique clinics" and concierge medicine.

Is this really what we want? A single payer, socialist society?

Free enterprise, entrepreneurship, and competition are what makes medicine in the US great. We must carefully consider the impacts that the decisions currently being made in Washington concerning our healthcare may ultimately affect our freedom. The time to get involved is now. Let your voice be heard. Advocate for your patients and your family. Let's get back to practicing the "art" of medicine and re-focus on what matters most — the care of the person suffering with illness.

22

Controlling
the Costs of Innovation

In a controversial study released in 2014, Tufts University's Center for the Study of Drug Development[1] estimated that the cost to bring a new drug to market exceeds nearly 2.6 billion dollars. The Study,[2] which was 40% funded by industry has been criticized for over estimating these costs in favor of industry and misrepresenting some cost estimates. While we will not know fully the extent of the methodology of the study until later in 2015 when it is published in a peer reviewed journal, these preliminary findings were released in advance and have already begun to spur debate.

However, irrespective of these criticisms, I believe that the study does have merit and brings an important issue forward — *is the FDA stifling innovation with excessive fees and paper-work? Are smaller, less well-funded researchers/corporations unable to significantly contribute without partnering with big pharma? Who will ultimately bear the increased cost of drug development?*

Innovation is what has always made healthcare in the US great — it is what separates us from the rest of the world. For

---

[1] http://csdd.tufts.edu/

[2] http://csdd.tufts.edu/news/complete_story/pr_tufts_csdd_2014_cost_study

decades, the US has been able to attract talent from throughout the world and this has resulted in numerous "game changing" breakthroughs in medicine. Through continued development of new drugs, new technologies and new ways to better treat disease, we are able to improve outcomes and reduce death from preventable disease. The US has always been a place where others from around the world have come to incubate and grow ideas. Now, it appears that innovation must come at a substantial cost — the increasing capital required for drug development as well as taxes on medical device companies only serve to squeeze out the "small guys with big ideas" and limit our ability to continue to produce new, more effective therapies and cures. In addition, these additional costs to the pharmaceutical industry are not simply added to their bottom line — they are pushed on to the healthcare consumer as well as Federally funded healthcare plans. Ultimately, the taxpayer bears the brunt of the increased cost.

In today's regulatory environment, it has become clear to many of us that the FDA has significantly hampered the development of new technologies in the US. We need only to look as far as our colleagues in Europe to see proof — for decades, nearly all new devices and drugs often get approval in Europe months — if not years — ahead of approval in the US. The science behind these drugs and devices remains rigorous but regulation and costs in the US market results in much of the early work occurring in the EU. While the FDA does employ expert physician lead advisory panels, the agency may or may not listen to the panel's advice.

The process of drug development is long and arduous. Government regulation, politics and greed have served to make it even more difficult. Physicians in academic medicine, scientists, pharmacologists and leaders in industry have learned to partner and share ideas in order to bring basic science principles from the bench to the bedside — ultimately translating ideas into cures. Collaboration is critical to success but it is not always easy to achieve. Certainly, big pharma is in place to make profits and increase market share. But as costs increase, many drug makers are putting less and less profit back into research and development. Growth can become stagnant and new ideas may never reach the bench or bedside. Federally funded research — such as National Institutes of Health (NIH) grants — face big cuts and budgets are often embroiled in political battles. Legislators use research dollars as bargaining chips and fund projects that appeal only to a particular interest group or a group of favored donors. Politics have no place in the funding of important medical research. Holding science hostage for an additional amendment or tag along to a bill only serves to delay important work that could potentially change a patient's life.

We must find a better way to promote medical innovation and reward research. *We must* find better ways to choose the most promising projects for funding. *We must* be good stewards of the R & D dollar and make every single investment count. *We must* remember exactly WHY research is necessary at all ...

As with most things in medicine, we must always pause and remember to focus on the *patient.* Advocating for the patient suffering with disease is the reason most of us became involved in medicine in the first place. Whether the study from Tufts overestimates the cost of development or not, it should still serve as a wake up call to us all. We must work to control the cost of developing new therapies — *we must* limit excessive taxation, *we must* promote entrepreneurship and begin to fix the current system of FDA approval for new therapies. *We must* separate politics from medicine and streamline processes — eliminate paperwork and promote efficiency — if we are to continue to lead the world in medical innovation. *We must* continue to make room for the "small guy with the big ideas" — if we do not — ultimately it will be our patients that suffer in the end.

23

"Veritas", Ivy and the Affordable Care Act: What is Good for the Goose May Now NOT be Good for the Gander at Harvard

Prominent academics within the prestigious Harvard University department of Economics have long been vocal supporters of President Obama and his Affordable Care Act (ACA) legislation. In fact, many Harvard professors helped develop some of the concepts that were utilized in the drafting of the ACA. Often vocal in the media, as well as in academic meetings, these professors waxed poetic about the need for reform and how cost sharing was the key to success. They argued that those who were healthy and could have little potential healthcare costs attributed to them would be needed to fund the elderly and those with chronic disease.

During the debates over the ACA in Congress, these professors were frequently seen (and heard) touting the legislation as a fiscally responsible way to provide affordable care to all Americans. Many of these academics received promotions and increased notoriety within their disciplines due to their participation in the development of the ACA as well as assisting the bill through the legislative process. The current Provost, Dr. Alan Garber, (not to be confused with Massachusetts Institute of Technology's (MIT) Gruber), was part of a group of economists who sent letters to the President in the early days of the ACA praising certain aspects of the bill such as "cost sharing" and the Cadillac tax applied to the best plans. These economists carefully examined multiple theoretical models and claimed that the legislation would certainly solve the fiscal problems of healthcare in the US today.

But we didn't mean to apply the law to us?

My, how things have changed! In early 2015, as reported in the *New York Times*,[1] these same Harvard faculty began to create an uproar as they watched their own healthcare plans completely overhauled. Rather than being allowed to maintain their long-time, low-cost (out-of-pocket) plans, the university has now implemented healthcare coverage that is consistent with the provisions in the ACA. Now there are more up-front, out-of-pocket expenses for basic insurance plans and the Cadillac plans are much more expensive. Interestingly, the very same academics who once touted the glories of the current ACA legislation in front of Congress are now taking a BIG step back.

During a faculty meeting the vast majority of Harvard professors voted to *oppose* the changes in the Harvard health plan that would require them to pay more for their *own* healthcare — all changes that are consistent with the plans they pitched before Congress just years before.

How *dare* Harvard adjust *their own* benefits and how *dare* the University actually expect *them* to be a part of a new ACA influenced healthcare plan at Harvard???

This type of attitude is even more prevalent among lawmakers in both the White House and in Congress. Members of Congress

---

[1] http://www.nytimes.com/2015/01/06/us/health-care-fixes-backed-by-harvards-experts-now-roil-its-faculty.html?ref=health

as well as the President and all staffers are EXEMPT from the individual mandate. This type of paternalistic governance is what is wrong with Washington today. Many Democrats seem to have taken the attitude that they were elected not to represent the people but rather to do what *they think is best* for their constituents. In an era when the ACA is wildly unpopular, many politicians continue to refuse to believe that changes to the legislation should be made.

If the ACA is such a great thing, why then do those who designed it and legislated it refuse to participate?

1. **The President and His Legacy:** The President continues to see the ACA as his legacy. In spite of plummeting approval numbers and a negative referendum on his failed policies during the 2014 midterm elections, Obama refuses to examine the numerous issues associated with the healthcare law and does not appear to have any willingness to compromise on amending the act. Unfortunately, Obama's pursuit of his legacy appears to trump sensible bipartisan negotiations and will severely limit Washington's ability to actually *govern.*

2. **Paternal Governance:** Currently, many in power feel as though they know what is "best" for the rest of us. Rather than represent a constituency, many of our leaders actually believe that the American people are incapable of making sound decisions for themselves and their own healthcare. The "Big Brother" knows best attitude continues to alienate millions of voting Americans. Interestingly, when those that helped craft the legislation (i.e. the now disgruntled Harvard economics professors) are subjected to the law that they supported, the outlook quickly changes.

3. **Partisan Politics:** Our country is now more divided politically than ever before. Relationships in Washington are so polarized that compromise will be difficult to achieve. Our elected government is divided with the President refusing to even consider bills that are put forward — instead he threatens vetoes in advance on any bills that address issues concerning the reform of the ACA.

So, what's next?

As a country we must begin to deal with the issue of healthcare in a more productive and collaborative way. Politics as usual will result in another two years, the decline in both the quality and affordability of the American healthcare system. We must hold Washington accountable and the Obama administration MUST begin to work with Congressional leaders to find workable, effective solutions to the mountain of problems that has been created by the poorly thoughtout and recklessly implemented ACA legislation. And, those at Harvard (as well as those in Washington) should have to live with the same healthcare insurance programs that are mandated for the rest of us — no exemptions.

24

Healthcare Industry CEOs and the Cost of Care: Too Many Men (and Women) in Black (Suits)?

Healthcare reform is a reality. The Affordable Care Act (ACA) and its associated mandates have forever changed the landscape of medicine in the US today. The Obama administration touts the goals of reform as providing affordable, cost-effective, high-quality care for all Americans. Certainly these are noble and lofty goals — but have we completely *missed the mark*? Today, many remain uninsured and the majority that have signed up for the exchanges are simply those who have lost their healthcare coverage from other providers. Healthcare costs in the US remain above those of all other industrialized countries while physician salaries in the US continue to fall. Even though the US spends more dollars-per-capita on healthcare than any other country on earth, our outcomes, when compared to other nations remain mediocre at best.

What about cost? Who is actually delivering care?

Over the last 30 years, hospital administrators and CEOs have grown by 2,500% while physicians have grown by only a modest amount. In fact, according to the American Academy of Family Practice, there must be a 25% increase in primary care doctors over the next 10 years in order to keep pace with demand. Multiple independent surveys (published by the AAMC[1]) indicate a significant shortfall of all types of physicians nationally by the year 2020. As administrators and insurance company executives grow, hospital staff and services continue to be cut — nurses and doctors are asked to care for more patients with fewer resources. Executives continue to tout savings within their organizations and boards award these administrators with enormous financial bonuses.

Source: The Bureau of Labour Statistics (BLS) and Hammelstein/Wool handler.

Where are the doctors in all of this?

The short answer is that physicians are caring for patients and managing the piles of paperwork that the government and other healthcare organizations and executives have created for them. Doctors are now consumed with checking boxes, implementing EMRs and transitioning to a new coding system for billing — all while seeing increasing patient loads and meeting increasingly steep clinical demands.

In an article in the *New York Times*,[2] author Elisabeth Rosenthal spells out what many physicians have known for a very long time — the administrators and hospitals are the high wage earners — not the doctors. As the number of administrators continues to rise exponentially, many independent physicians and physician groups

---

[1] https://www.aamc.org/download/100598/data/
[2] http://www.nytimes.com/2014/05/18/sunday-review/doctors-salaries-are-not-the-big-cost.html?hp&rref=opinion&_r=1

are being driven to integrate with or leave practice altogether in order to remain fiscally viable. According to the *Times*, the salaries of many administrators and CEOs (in both the hospitals and the insurance industry) are outpacing salaries of both general practice physicians, surgeons and even most specialists. Astronomical wages such as those earned by Aetna's CEO (total package over 36 million dollars) and others are a big contributing factor to the trillions of dollars that we spend on healthcare each year. According to the *New York Times*, healthcare administrative costs make up nearly 30% of the total US healthcare bill. Obviously, large corporations and CEOs will argue that these wages are necessary to attract the best and brightest executives to the healthcare industry. What is there to attract the best and brightest scientists to medicine? Certainly altruism is a big part of what physicians are about but economic realities must still come into play when bright young students are choosing careers (while accumulating graduate and professional school debt at record paces).

Why then does it seem as though physicians are the only target for reform?

That answer is simple — hospital administrators and insurance company CEOs are well trained businessmen (and women) with MBAs from prestigious schools. They understand politics and how to effectively lobby. They have been actively involved in reform and have participated in discussions on Capitol Hill rather than watch the change happen around them. When costs are cut from the healthcare expenditures, they have made erudite moves — they have worked effectively to isolate themselves and their institutions from the cuts that are affecting the rest of the industry. While reimbursement for office visits and procedures falls to less than 50% through many of the exchanges and other government based programs such as Medicare and Medicaid, CEOs and hospital administrators continue to financially outpace their colleagues in other sectors of business.

As physicians, we must continue to focus on our patients and their well being. Individually, we must continue to provide outstanding, efficient, quality care to those who depend on us every single day. As a group, however, doctors must begin to work harder to influence those in Washington for change. While healthcare reform is essential and must be accomplished in a fiscally responsible way, it is my hope that those in a position to effect change will recognize that we must begin to better regulate and limit those in CEO and administrative positions in both the insurance and hospital industries. Just as we reduce the numbers of nurses on the floor to care for patients in order to save healthcare dollars, maybe we should eliminate a few Vice Presidents (VPs) with fancy offices on the top floors of our hospitals. Which one do you think will positively impact patients more — fewer nurses or fewer dark suits?

Part Five
Reform and the Future of Medicine

Introduction

Traditions are slow to change. The practice of medicine has been handed down from scholar to scholar for generations. While the science is continually evolving, the basic ways in which we care for patients and families remain constant. Care, compassion, empathy and the development of human relationships have been the cornerstone of exceptional medical care throughout the ages.

Reform has arrived and now the way in which medicine is practiced is changing. Doctors are asked to do more with less and are forced to spend more time with non-clinical activities. Administrative challenges such as Electronic Medical Records (EMR), "meaningful use" documentation and declining reimbursement have led to a great deal of physician discontent and burnout.

Moreover, the expanded pool of newly insured patients has resulted in a pending doctor shortage. Some blame the lack of training slots but others blame the unattractive practice environment on the declining numbers of physicians in training. While the numbers of "Medical Administrators" emerging from universities has increased by 3000% over the last 10 years, the numbers of newly minted doctors has remained relatively constant. The doctor shortage has resulted in expanded roles for nurses, nurse practitioners and other allied health professionals.

Declining reimbursement in concert with the increasing work-load (much of which is non-clinical) has resulted in widespread physician discontent. Physicians with specialties that crossover in expertise have resorted to turf battles within hospital systems in order to increase or protect reimbursement patterns. All of this has resulted in a relatively dysfunctional operation within many healthcare systems.

In this section, we explore each of these issues — how health-care reform has set medicine on a new path. These essays examine the impact of government-mandated change on the daily practice of medicine and how it may forever change the way in which patients interface with the medical system. While the future of medicine may look relatively bleak, it is my hope that we can "right the ship", and rewrite healthcare reform in a way that allows for a more sensible, patient focused delivery of care.

25

The Doctor Shortage
of Tomorrow: Fact or Fiction?

Today there is a great debate over the impact that the Affordable Care Act (ACA) may have on physician supply and demand. Dr. Scott Gottlieb and Dr. Ezekiel Emanuel, the architect of the ACA, have publicly stated and made the case in several Op Ed pieces that there will NOT be a physician shortage as a result of ACA. Both have extensive experience in policy and have held respected positions in government. Based on a projected need of nearly 90,000 more physicians by 2020, I have difficulty seeing how a shortage will not occur. The ACA has already demonstrated the ineptness of government to manage healthcare — the laughable website rollout, newly discovered "backend" issues with signups, inaccurate quotes and information and questionable security. Now, as the mandates are implemented, consumers are beginning to wonder where exactly they will be able to get care and who may be providing it...

How can there NOT be a physician shortage?

Using the Massachusetts healthcare plan as an example, Drs. Gottlieb and Emmanuel argue that the shortage predictions are flawed. However, Massachusetts is not at all representative of the entire

US — one cannot extrapolate the response in Massachusetts to the rural Midwest, or the deep South or sunny California. Moreover, the provisions and funding of the legislation in Massachusetts are very different from those in the ACA. (It's like comparing apples to oranges). They argue that the biggest driver of increased physician manpower needs is more related to an aging population rather than the impacts of Obamacare and the flood of new patients that are insured by either Medicaid or the ACA exchanges that are able to set reimbursement levels at new all-time lows. They state that the solution to shortage issues will come in the form of technology driven "remote medicine" and the use of non-physician extenders such as advanced practice nurses and physician assistants. Moreover, they go on to argue that the solution is NOT producing more doctors — rather it is getting those of us in current practice to become "more efficient".

Really? We are already doing more every day with much, much less than we have had in the past ...

As doctors often do in clinical practice, I respectfully disagree with their assessment. Obamacare will continue to flood the system with millions of newly insured patients — if they can effectively sign up and afford the likely increases in premiums that are inevitable. As evidenced by the current climate in California, many physicians will choose NOT to participate in the exchanges due to very poor reimbursement rates. Recent surveys in that state found that nearly 75% of doctors would not take the exchange insurance or Medicaid due to the fact that the exchange payments were far below the standard CMS Medicare rates. Many practices are unable to maintain autonomy as payments continue to decrease — many are being integrated into hospital systems. Overhead continues to increase in order to meet Federal requirements for electronic documentation and records as well as maintaining coding experts to keep up with the ever changing systems such as the newly minted ICD-10. The concept of a completely free-standing private practice will no longer exist within the next three years.

Whether in academic or private settings, all physician groups will be employees of health conglomerates.

What is ultimately going to drive the physician shortage and what are the potential solutions?

For starters ... I certainly do not have all the answers ... While I do agree that the aging population certainly presents a manpower challenge, I do not concede that this alone will be the driving force behind any potential physician shortage. Medicine is becoming less attractive for young bright students considering a career in healthcare. Training physicians is expensive — medical schools are pricey for potential students and post-graduate training (Internship, Residency and Fellowship) are costly for the academic centers where they learn. Financially, students may no longer be able to incur the significant debt (in the hundreds of thousands of dollars) that continues to accrue when attending medical school when the job prospects promise declining financial rewards. Once in practice, newly minted MDs will find that their hours are longer and the time that they spend with each patient will be more limited — increasing documentation requirements will result in more screen time and less time listening and bonding.

Physicians are essential to the delivery of care. However, I also recognize the vital role that physician extenders play in healthcare today (and will in the future). Nurse practitioners, physician assistants and pharmacists are critical in ensuring that patient care is optimized. These providers must work in concert with physicians — approaching the whole patient in a team-care model will ultimately improve outcomes. But, utilizing these allied health professionals in more independent and unsupervised roles as Drs. Gottlieb and Emmanuel suggest is reckless. Although well trained and expert in their scope of practice, these allied health professionals are not physicians — they have not completed the academic rigors of a four year medical school nor gained the experience of a three to eight year Residency and

Fellowship. Replacing doctors with other provider types will NOT eliminate the need for physicians and will NOT forestall the expected physician shortage as we move into 2014 and beyond. We must continue to work with physician extenders and other allied health professionals in order to meet the increasing demands of a busy medical practice — I do not advocate for the independent practice that is currently being considered in many states.

Remote medicine, telemedicine and remote monitoring are certainly complementary and extremely valuable in providing care. In fact, as Drs. Gottlieb and Emanuel suggest, these modalities may reduce the number of doctor visits and may play a major role in prevention. While I am a real advocate for utilizing technology to engage patients and facilitate care, face to face interactions between doctor and patient must still be a part of the process. We cannot rely on computers and other electronic devices in isolation — they can, however, enhance the delivery of care when carefully included in a comprehensive treatment plan.

Are we simply losing our way as medicine remains in crisis ...

Ultimately, time will certainly determine the state of physician supply. If we remain on our current course and continue to fund and implement (albeit haphazardly) the provisions of the ACA, we will ultimately see the fallout of a significant physician shortage. Long lines, significant wait times and scarcity of both newly trained primary care and specialty doctors will become reality. Medicine in our country is at a crossroads. We must continue to advocate for our patients and protect our right to practice our noble profession in a way that provides the best possible outcomes for our patients today and in the future.

26

More (or less) Hope and Change (for the worse) in Healthcare: Are Doctor Shortages Really All Due to Training Bottlenecks?

There is no doubt that Affordable Care Act (ACA) has changed the landscape of medicine in the US. Now, private practice is becoming a thing of the past. Financial pressures, increasing regulatory requirements, electronic medical records and outrageously complex coding systems are forcing longtime private physicians to enter into agreements with academic centers and large hospital systems in order to survive. As a result, medicine today is more about increasing patient volumes, completing reams of paperwork and administrative duties than it is about interacting with patients and providing superior care. The American Academy of Family Physicians[1] estimates that there will be a significant shortage of primary care physicians in the next

---

[1]http://www.aafp.org/news/practice-professional-issues/20121114workforceneeds.html

several years unless we increase the number of primary care trainees by more than 25% over the same time period. In fact, the
AAFP suggests that the primary care workforce must increase to
260K physicians by the year 2025 — which translates to an additional 52K primary care doctors.

Given the need for more physicians and the looming shortage
(particularly in primary care), many analysts have suggested that
the reason for the shortage is the lack of training slots in primary
care. The ACA will add an additional 32 million patients to the
pool of insured and primary care doctors will be at a premium.
There are many conflicting opinions as to the reason for the doctor
shortage. Some, including the *New York Times* editorial board,
believe that the shortage is all about an imbalance between
Residency training slots and medical school graduates and can be
easily corrected by federal funding of a larger number of training
positions. However, I think that the issue is much more complex
and the solution is far from simple.

Primary care is an incredibly challenging specialty and requires
a broad knowledge of much of medicine. Reimbursements for
primary care work continue to lag and physicians are now spending more time with administrative duties than they are with
patients. I do not believe that the so-called post graduate training
"bottleneck" will come into play. I would suggest that many primary care training slots will go unfilled over the next 5–10 years
even without increasing the numbers of available positions.
Increasing training slots for primary care specialties may do
nothing to alleviate shortages if there are no students who wish to
train. While medical school enrollments have increased over the
last decade, much of this increased enrollment may be due to a lack
of jobs available to recent college graduates. Moreover, as the ACA
continues to evolve, physicians are now realizing lower compen-
sation rates, increased work hours, more administrative duties
and LESS time spent caring for patients. Many physicians are
forced to double the number of patients seen in a clinic day —
resulting in less than 10 minutes per patient — in order to meet

overhead and practice expenses. In a separate article in the *New York Times*,[2] author and cardiologist Sandeep Jauhar discusses the increased patient loads and subsequent higher rates of diagnostic testing that is required in order to make sure that nothing is missed ultimately increasing the cost of care. Defensive medicine, excessive testing and fears of litigation promote more costly care.

For most of those who have entered medicine, the attraction to the profession is all about the doctor–patient interaction and the time spent caring for others. I would argue that the primary care shortage (and likely specialist shortage) will worsen in the future. Many bright minds will likely forego medicine in order to pursue other less government-regulated careers. In addition, many qualified primary care physicians will opt out of the ACA system and enter into the rapidly growing concierge care practice model. The answer to the physician shortage may be more political than not — politicians must realize that laws and mandates only work if you have citizens willing to devote their time, energy and talents to the practice of medicine. Going forward, more consideration must be given to physician quality of life and autonomy must be maintained. In order to make healthcare reform sustainable, those in power must work with those of us "in the trenches" and create policies that are in the best interest of the patient, the physician and the nation as a whole. Cutting costs must be approached from multiple angles — not simply reducing the size of the physician paycheck.

Medicine remains a noble profession. Those of us that do continue to practice medicine are privileged to serve others and provide outstanding care. In order to continue to advance, we must continue to attract bright young minds who are willing to put patients and their needs above their own — at all costs.

---

[2] http://www.nytimes.com/2014/07/21/opinion/busy-doctors-wasteful-spending.html

I think that there is still HOPE to save medicine in the US. It is my HOPE that our government will soon realize that in order to continue to propagate a workforce of competent, caring physicians we must provide time for physicians to do what they do best — bond with patients and treat disease (as opposed to typing into a computer screen and filling out endless reams of electronic paperwork). It is my HOPE that those physicians in training that will follow in my generation's footsteps will realize the satisfaction that comes from impacting the health and lives of patients over time. It is my HOPE that the ART of medicine can be saved before it is too late.

27

Doctors Punching Time Clocks: The Impact of Reform

Much debate remains around the concept of healthcare reform in the US today. Almost all of us agree that our current system is broken and in need of an overhaul. However, there are trends in the healthcare market that are increasingly troubling.

Due to changes in reimbursement, demands for Electronic Medical Records, documentation changes related to International Classification of Diseases — 10 the revision (ICD-10) coding requirements and federally mandated quality measures, physicians can no longer afford to remain independent. All of these changes require more work and additional office personnel. Based on projections made by healthcare analysts, over 90% of cardiology practices will have "integrated" or assimilated (reference the Borg from *Star Trek*)[1] with hospital systems by the year 2016. Overall, it is estimated that over 50% of all types of physician practices will be hospital-owned in the next year. The loss of the traditional physician-owned private practice will forever change the medical marketplace. As a medical resident, we were always taught that the work day was done, when all the work was

---

[1] http://en.wikipedia.org/wiki/Borg_(Star_Trek)

done — that translated into long hours and little rest. These residency work habits follow most physicians into practice and rarely do physicians have regular work hours. It is not uncommon to start before dawn and complete chart work and dictation late into the night. If market trends continue along the path of integration and assimilation of individual practices by hospital systems we are going to begin to develop a very different culture of healthcare delivery where physicians may ultimately become hourly employees who "clock in and clock out" at the end of a shift.

Several scholars have examined the idea of doctors who "clock in and clock out" as hospital employees rather than small business owners. One particular opinion piece published in the *Wall Street Journal* and written by Scott Gottlieb, is quite sobering. In his Op Ed piece, Mr. Gottlieb correctly highlights some of the issues associated with doctors as employees. First of all, the acquisition of practices and physicians by hospital systems is often based on competitive advantage and market share increases in a particular area rather than on providing the best quality care. Hospital systems leverage facilities, salaries and some cleverly push competitors out of the market by creating monopolies of care. However, a larger problem is that there are some data that suggest that when doctors are employed by hospital systems, productivity actually declines. When in practice and financially invested in the success of one's own practice or organization, physicians tend to work longer hours and squeeze in more procedures, office visits and phone calls. However, when physicians become employees, productivity decreases. There are many reasons for the decreased productivity including the way in which physician work is actually measured and calculated by hospitals (based on Medicare rules). Physician work, measured in relative value units (RVUs) arbitrarily assigns numerical values to tasks that are commonly performed in medicine. Not all agree that these assigned values are fair and equitable.

Ultimately we must decrease cost in healthcare. Obamacare was crafted in order to provide access to care for all Americans

AND to lower costs. Unfortunately, Mr. Gottlieb and I both agree that the pending healthcare reforms may actually increase costs in the long run. The initial result of the reform legislation has been the trend of hospital acquisition of practices — and the resulting decrease in productivity. So, it is not a great leap to assume that as more physicians become employees who punch a time clock, the actual cost of care will increase substantially.

We must continue to work together to provide better solutions for our healthcare dilemma. All players must be involved in crafting reform — physicians, politicians, hospitals, insurers, pharma and industry. We cannot focus on one group and not the others. The ultimate solution for healthcare delivery in the US will be the result of collaboration and regulation of all pieces of the healthcare puzzle.

28

The Advantages of Team Approaches to Patient Care: Extending NOT Replacing Physician Care

Let me start by stating that I am a supporter of team approaches to medical care. Data from numerous observational trials has shown that patient outcomes are improved when a diverse group of healthcare providers work together to coordinate overall patient care. In my practice, we rely heavily on the excellent care provided by both physician assistants as well as nurse practitioners both in the hospital and in the clinics. These physician extenders are essential to coordinating admissions, evaluations, testing and treatments.

Many in the mainstream media, including *Wall Street Journal* columnist Laura Landro have examined the new push for team-based care in today's healthcare market. There are numerous advantages to the team based approach. Patients benefit from the more intensive one-on-one time that they are afforded with nutritionists, pharmacists, nurses and other advanced practitioners. In previous decades, most of this work was solely the responsibility of the physician. However, increasing demands for documentation and electronic paperwork have begun to consume physician time.

While the Affordable Care Act (ACA) promises to flood primary care offices with even more patients, physicians are scrambling to perform all of the duties that are currently required of them (with more government mandates on the horizon). Most of my colleagues prefer to focus on patient care (rather than administrative paperwork and government mandates) but are often frustrated by how little time they have to interact with their patients. Managing chronic disease is a process and requires numerous "touch points" with the patient in order to be successful. In reality, as a cardiologist, I am able to see most of my stable patients only once a quarter — unless they have an acute event or decompensation.

It is clear that patients now are living with more complex diseases and that we have far more advanced therapies to treat them with. Many of these therapies rely on strict patient compliance and on patients having a thorough understanding of their disease process and its management. For instance, a patient with Congestive Heart Failure (CHF) may need to be able to interpret daily weights and adjust diuretic dosing accordingly in order to prevent hospitalization from a more serious CHF exacerbation. Now, rather than see a physician for medication discussions every three months, a patient can make an appointment with a Pharmacist in our office and see them on a more frequent basis to discuss concerns over efficacy or side effects of their medical regimen. In our experience, this has improved patient compliance and improved metrics such as blood pressure control and time spent in the therapeutic range for chronic anticoagulation patients. Other primary care physicians report similar results when managing diabetes *via* frequent nurse educator or NP visits — patients seem to have more consistent control and better glycated hemoglobin (HbA1C) results when they have more frequent touch points.

While a team approach is quite effective, each team must have a leader. The team leader must be experienced and well trained. While physician extenders do receive extensive training in a two to four year program, nothing replaces the years of experience that MDs obtain during residency. In order to maintain a high standard of patient care, these teams must still be led by physicians. With the cost cutting efforts and the changes that are occurring in healthcare due to the ACA, I am concerned that hospital administrators and government bureaucrats will ultimately attempt to replace physicians with other healthcare providers in the interest of curtailing costs. Physicians are trained in real-life patient care scenarios over a period of years — many residencies last from three to ten years depending on specialty. The experiences of call nights and handling real-time emergencies over a period of years (under the supervision of more experienced attending physicians) cannot be undervalued. My experiences during my seven years of postgraduate training at both the University of Virginia and Duke University Medical Center certainly shaped my clinical judgement and certainly sharpened my diagnostic abilities — I call on these experiences even today when faced with complex cases. Efforts to replace physicians with other healthcare professionals with less intensive training may ultimately harm patient care.

Patient care comes first — I believe that a team based approach is essential to optimizing outcomes. *We must all work together* — nurses, NPs, PAs, pharmacists, nutritionists, and MDs — in order to provide the best possible patient centered care. However, we must not attempt to replace physicians and the experience that they bring to the clinical arena in the interest of cost containment. While balancing cost and optimal care is a slippery slope, we must always *focus on the patient* — nothing can or should replace the doctor–patient relationship — we must all work together to preserve the core principles of our noble profession and put our patients first.

29

The Electronic Medical Record Mandate and Managing Fraud: More Government Ineptness?

The Obama administration has clearly mandated that Electronic Medical Records (EMR) will be necessary in order to comply with Federal regulations for reimbursement for both hospitals and physicians. The transition to EMR is an important step towards streamlining patient care — however, the current implementation of EMR is fraught with complications, workflow issues and system wide "bugs". At this point in the US there are numerous EMR systems and no absolute standard which continues to make communication between different hospital systems and physicians difficult at times. I realize that the EMR mandate has spanned more than one administration and let me state at the very outset that I am 100% FOR the implementation of an EMR system. However, I would like to see the transition done in a stepwise, intelligent way that allows for universal portability within the US. Moreover, the EMR should be electronically available to all patients *via* smartphone and tablet download from the mysterious (and hopefully secure) "cloud".

The EMR when properly managed can provide detailed notes that are easily applied to templates for billing Medicare and Medicaid documentation (it allows MDs to correctly bill the level of service based on comparison of the patient's newly created chart-note to standards for required components). However, the time involved in documenting *via* EMR (especially in the transition phase in a busy practice) can be overwhelming. Physicians and other providers are already overwhelmed with offices full of patients — longer hours, more appointments and loads of new paperwork. The Affordable Care Act (ACA) promises to add loads of newly insured sick patients to the practice workload. Add to that a cumbersome computer system and it is likely that errors will occur.

Our own Department of Justice has now begun to focus on EMR fraud activities. The Office of Inspector General (OIG) for Department of Health and Human Services (HHS) has released several reports[1] warning of the potential widespread fraud and abuse occurring as a result of EMR implementation. The warning specifically cites a lack of oversight and safeguards in the Federal government to prevent these from occurring. The government has already spent nearly 22 billion dollars on the push for conversion from paper to EMR in the US (sounds familiar? rapid roll out of new technology without proper evaluation).

According to several reports, the central issue with the EMR and potential fraud has to do with the lack of regulations surrounding the common practice of "copy and paste" known as "cloning". For many physicians, the ability to cut and paste data and information from one place to another in a note or within a patient's particular chart can significantly improve efficiency and reduce the amount of time that is spent inputting redundant data into a patient's record. Critics of this practice, including the OIG, suggest that in many cases the importation of data from note to note or chart to chart results in "overbilling" for services that were

---

[1]http://oig.hhs.gov/oei/reports/oei-01-11-00571.pdf

not in fact rendered. For example, if a chart note from a follow-up visit of moderate complexity is "cloned" with data from a previous visit where the level of service was more extensive than the current visit, then charges may be filed for a level of complexity that was not, in fact, provided. The OIG statement goes on to warn that their "level of involvement in EMR cases [will] increase" and that dealing with documentation "fraud" *via* cloning in EMR will become a "top priority". In a survey[2] conducted by HHS and released in a previous report, the OIG found that very few hospitals and medical practices have any guidelines or restrictions on "cloning" notes for documentation.

Once again, in my opinion, our government has missed its mark. Instead of carefully creating a universally acceptable and streamlined EMR that allows for responsible and efficient data entry AND migration of data to subsequent encounters, federal regulators have issued yet another mandate without a clear vision of its implications. As I stated earlier, I believe EMR is vital for patient information management and will ultimately help us provide more streamlined care that is evidence based. Unfortunately, the current EMR systems that are in place do not place a priority on ease of use, efficiency or portability. Although I am sure that there is some intentional documentation fraud occurring, I would suggest that the majority of physicians and other providers are simply trying to "get the job done" and move on to more important patient care activities. EMR documentation can be slow and arduous. During transition phases, many providers report two to three extra hours added to their days for documentation activities. No physician wants to continually take a practice laptop home in order to finish entering EMR notes during family time night after night. Cloning data is a simple way to carry over information such as medication lists, past medical histories and other information in order to improve efficiency while at the same time providing adequate documentation. As

---

[2]https://oig.hhs.gov/oei/reports/oei-01-11-00570.pdf

with most things, this type of data migration is easy to abuse if physicians do not pay special attention to ensure that the migrated data is both accurate and representative of the work that was performed.

As the current administration has clearly demonstrated with the rollout of the ACA, as well as with the new ICD-10 coding system[3] and the EMR mandates, sweeping reform that is rushed to completion without a full understanding of its implications is doomed to fail. Putting politics and power ahead of good sense has resulted in increased cost for these government mandated programs. As a nation we must certainly work to prevent fraud and abuse as part of our efforts to curtail healthcare costs. However, as we initiate reforms, we must do a much better job of anticipating issues with new technologies and work to deal with them on the front end — if we do not, we can expect costs to continue to rise.

---

[3] http://drkevincampbellmd.wordpress.com/2013/12/30/the-next-government-based-healthcare-debacle-coding-for-orca-bites/

30

Turf Battles and Collateral Damage: Are We Really Putting the Patient First?

Turf battles are nothing new in medicine. In the last year, a very public battle occurred between dermatologists and AHPs (Allied Health Professionals) over the performance of dermatologic procedures. As independent NPs (Nurse Practitioners) and PAs (Physician Assistants) begin to bill for more and more procedures (thus potentially taking revenue away from board certified dermatologists) specialists are beginning to argue that the AHPs are practicing beyond their scope of practice. According to the *Journal of the American Medical Association*,[1] nearly five million dermatological procedures were performed by NPs and PAs last year — this has dermatologists seeking practice limits — ostensibly to protect "bread and butter" revenue streams from biopsies, skin tag removals and other common office based interventions.

First of all I want to say that AHPs are essential to providing care in the era of the Affordable Care Act (ACA). NPs and PAs are able to help meet the needs of underserved areas and do a remarkable job complementing the care of the physicians with whom they

---

[1] http://archderm.jamanetwork.com/article.aspx?articleid=1895673

work. With the rapidly expanded pool of newly insured, as well as the increase in administrative tasks (electronic documentation) assigned to physicians, AHPs must help fill in the gaps and ensure that all patients have access to care. In my practice we are fortunate to have many well qualified AHPs who assist us in the care of our patients both in the hospital as well as in the office.

We must remember, however, that physicians and AHPs have very different training. Each professional possesses a unique set of skills and each skill set can complement the others. Many of us in specialty areas spend nearly a decade in post MD training programs and learn how to care for patients through rigorous, round the clock shifts during our Residency and Fellowship years. In addition, we spend countless hours performing specialized procedures over this time and are closely supervised by senior staff. Most AHPs, in contrast, do not spend time in lengthy residencies and often have limited exposure to specialized procedures. Turf battles have existed for decades and are certainly not limited to Dermatology — nor or they limited to MDs versus AHPs. In cardiology in the late 1990s, for instance, we struggled in turf battles with Radiology over the performance of Peripheral Vascular Interventions. In many areas, these battles resulted in limited availability of specialized staff to patients and a lack of integrated care. Ultimately, the patients were the ones who suffered.

Fortunately, in the University of North Carolina (UNC) Healthcare system where I work (as well as others across the country) we have taken a very different approach. After observing inefficiencies and redundancy in the system, several years ago our leadership (under the direction of Dr. Cam Patterson) decided to make a change. The UNC Heart and Vascular Center[2] was created — vascular surgeons, cardiologists, interventional radiologists, and cardiothoracic surgeons — all working under one cooperative umbrella. Patients are now discussed and treated with a multidisciplinary approach — electrophysiologists

---

[2]http://www.uncheartandvascular.org/

and cardiothoracic surgeons perform hybrid Atrial Fibrillation ablation procedures, vascular surgeons and interventional cardiologists discuss the best way to approach a patient with carotid disease — all working together to produce the BEST outcome for each individual patient. We have seen patient satisfaction scores improve and we have noted that access to multiple specialty consultations has become much easier to achieve in a timely fashion. Most importantly, communication among different specialties has significantly improved.

Unfortunately, with the advent of the ACA and decreasing reimbursement I suspect that turf battles will continue. Financial pressures have become overwhelming for many practices and the days of the private practice are limited — more and more groups will continue to "integrate" with large hospital systems in the coming years. Specialists such as dermatologists and others will continue to (rightly so) protect procedures that provide a revenue stream in order to remain financially viable. However, I believe that our time will be better spent by working together to improve efficiency of care, quality of care and integration of care. NPs and PAs are going to be a critical component to healthcare delivery as we continue to adapt to the new (and ever changing) ACA mandates. We must put patients FIRST — turf battles and squabbles amongst healthcare providers will only limit our ability to provide outstanding, efficient care. Let's put the most qualified person in the procedure room — and make sure that ultimately patients get exactly what they need.

Index

ACA Exchange insurance, 59
access issues, 82
access to care, 43, 93
Accreditation Council for Graduate
  Medical Education (ACGME),
  69
administrators, 87
Affordable Care Act (ACA), 3, 7,
  9, 13, 21, 23, 25, 34, 38, 41, 45,
  53, 59, 62, 73, 74, 79,83,, 87,
  89, 93, 105, 109, 117, 121, 130,
  134, 137
AHPs (Allied Health Professionals),
  137
American Academy of Family
  Physicians, 121
American Academy of Family
  Practice, 110
American College of Cardiology
  (ACC), 34
American Medical Association,
  90
Apple, 14
  Apple Watch, 15
  iOS 8, 14
  iPad, 17, 18, 20
  iPhone 6, 14

art of medicine, 56, 71
Association of American Medical
  Colleges (AAMC), 19, 110
autonomy, 42

Big Brother, 10
big pharma, 28, 102
bureaucrats, 15
burnout, 32, 33, 41, 42, 50, 70

Center for Medicare and Medicaid
  Services (CMS), 53, 98
Centers for Disease Control
  (CDC), 9
choice, 61, 62, 91
chronic lymphocytic leukemia
  (CLL), 26
CMS Medicare, 118
collaboration, 102
communication, 80
competition, 99
concierge medicine, 42
Congestive Heart Failure (CHF),
  81, 130
Congress, 23
cost, 8, 25
cost-effective, 109